MILK

An Intimate History of Breastfeeding

JOANNA WOLFARTH

T0343558

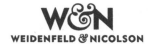

WEIDENFELD & NICOLSON

First published in Great Britain in 2023 by Weidenfeld & Nicolson
This paperback edition first published in Great Britain in 2024 by
Weidenfeld & Nicolson,
an imprint of The Orion Publishing Group Ltd
Carmelite House, 50 Victoria Embankment
London EC4Y 0DZ

An Hachette UK Company

1 3 5 7 9 10 8 6 4 2

A CIP catalogue record for this book is
available from the British Library.

ISBN (Mass Market Paperback) 978 1 4746 2323 0
ISBN (eBook) 978 1 4746 2324 7
ISBN (Audio) 978 1 4746 2325 4

Typeset by Input Data Services Ltd, Bridgwater, Somerset

Printed and bound in Great Britain by Clays Ltd, Elcograf S.p.A.

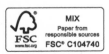

www.weidenfeldandnicolson.co.uk
www.orionbooks.co.uk

For FWS

CONTENTS

CONTENTS

There is always within her at least a little of that good mother's milk. She writes in white ink.

Hélène Cixous

INTRODUCTION

Milk is elemental. It is the first thing we look for at birth and, for most, it is the first substance to touch our tongues after we enter the world. It is the promise of nourishment, of care, of life. Milk is hope. In Exodus, God describes the Promised Land to Moses as 'flowing with milk and honey', life-giving liquids that imply sweetness and sex. Milk synonymous with fertility and, apparently, springing from nothing.

But we know otherwise. Milk is made, prepared and delivered. It is a baby at the breast, compelling the body to produce more, it is a person patiently expressing milk with a breast pump, a parent carefully measuring spoonfuls of formula as they wait for the kettle to boil, or a mother with donor breast milk that she will feed to her baby using a tube attached to her nipple. It is the transfer of nutrition.

But milk is so much more.

Milk is about bodies, our own and those of others. Milk is emotional. It is where our senses and desires first mingle. There is pleasure to be gained from sucking and from satisfying hunger, from the sensation of milk running down the throat. But there is also the pain of denial, of unmet needs, of being unlatched. We may not remember our infancy, but perhaps those memories are stored somewhere deep within our bones. Pause for a moment and you may feel that warmth of memory in your body.

Milk is relational. There is reciprocal touch, smell, taste, sound and eye contact. Whether it comes from a breast or a bottle, milk offers us our first intersubjective experiences. Between a caregiver and baby, but also with partners and families, communities and governments. Infant-feeding practices are as cultural as they are instinctual and can define, alter and challenge a multitude of identities and relationships. Milk is not only about survival; it is also about socialisation.

Milk structures our worlds. According to one linguist, *mama* derives from the nasal murmur made when the lips are satisfyingly pressed against a breast or bottle.[1] That same sound is eventually reproduced as babbling speech to communicate desire, for milk, for comfort. Across disparate language groups the primary caregiver's name derives from the syllables of that soft murmur. I was *mama* until I became *mummy*. My friend in Cambodia is *mak*, while my Sri Lankan friend was *amma*. And at first, we were all indistinguishable from sustenance.

There are etymological wormholes to get lost in but, in essence, to mother is to nurture. *Mother* is not a fixed and stable identity. Instead, like *love*, it is both a noun and a verb. In this book I use a variety of terms for those who engage in 'motherwork': doing, caring, nurturing, sacrificing, subsuming oneself in order to let another thrive.[2] Although the term motherwork maintains the gender binary that sadly still underpins child-rearing, I know that not only is mothering not restricted to a gestational or birthing body, it must also include trans and non-binary parents, as well as adoptive parents. And nor is a more expansive definition of 'mother' simply a contemporary phenomenon. For example, in written sources from ancient Mesopotamia, the closest translation to the English definition of mother is *ummu*. Sources demonstrate that those who carried out caregiving duties associated with being a guardian – such as wet-nursing – were afforded this title.[3] A feeding body isn't always the same body that gave birth to the infant. A feeding or birthing body may not belong to a woman. Lately there has been much made of the use of inclusive language, particularly in perinatal services in the UK, but to paraphrase Shon Faye, author of *The Transgender Issue*, true inclusivity and embracing the beautiful diversity in parenting can only be of benefit to all individuals.

Milk is between binaries.

My relationship with milk is my earliest memory. I'm standing in my red fleece nightdress next to the rocking chair, my teddy tucked under an arm, bare feet on floorboards. The house is dark and quiet. But here my mother sits in the glow of a reading lamp, my baby brother making gentle snuffles and grunts as he nurses. She draws me closer into the warmth of her body with her free arm and I ask her about the words in the glossy magazine that's opened across her lap. Maybe I don't say 'words'. Maybe I ask how to draw letters or what the black patterns mean. This is my earliest memory, but also a story my mother likes to tell often, and it is impossible to disentangle my own recollections from her retellings. But what I do know for certain is that Mum passes me a biro and helps me write my first letters in the margins of that magazine, as my brother softly gulps down her milk. J-o-a-n-n-a – there I am. Outside, the apple blossom falls silently from the trees and, in a few hours, we'll open the curtains to find the pavements carpeted white.

As a breastfed baby myself, when I had my own children I assumed breastfeeding would come easily. I had grown up aware of the 'breast is best' campaign that the

UK government initiated in 1999, and I knew all about the benefits of breast milk. And, from the little I knew about the practicalities of breastfeeding, I thought that it would be enough to have breasts and the desire to feed. Simple, if not always easy. I respected those who chose to bottle-feed – and do so now more than ever – but it just wasn't how I envisaged my motherhood. Whenever I idly pictured myself as a new mother, I saw it almost exactly as Renoir had pictured his wife, Aline Charigot, in his 1885 portrait *Maternité*. It was painted the year Charigot gave birth to their first child, a boy named Pierre. Such a serene, aspirational picture of motherhood and breastfeeding. Charigot is perched on a log, one foot resting on a stone. Her cheeks are rosy and her hair hangs loose below her hat as she unselfconsciously feeds her baby. Her milk has converted into rolls of fat on the baby's legs, which he kicks in the air in order to investigate his own foot. Heavy eyelids betray exhaustion, yet Charigot appears wholesome and at ease. I craved that abundance.

When our time came, it's true that we had times when the joy I experienced was transcendent. But there are also jagged edges to those memories.

Breastfeeding wasn't as I'd expected.

Within three weeks of my son's birth, I knew something wasn't right. Yes, a little nipple pain at first is to be expected and yes, it is very common and quite normal for babies to lose a little birth weight, but, body battered and mind addled, all I could think was: *something is wrong*. I went to the local, free breastfeeding support café, where, over a hot cup of tea, I was told that he was feeding well. But it continued to hurt, and the baby seemed to be in great distress most of the time and, more alarmingly, seemed to stop putting weight on. Lack of serious investment in perinatal services left us going between peer supporters, GP, midwives and health visitors, without the true, joined-up support new parents desperately need. We had no idea what was normal and so, on the advice of a health visitor, I took him to the GP to see if he had reflux. The GP was kind and told me about his own small children. He assured me I had nothing to worry about. But he didn't weigh the baby and I left feeling like the cliché of a new mother, unnecessarily worried and anxious.

On a bright Sunday afternoon one week later, our midwife sent us to A&E and we were admitted overnight. My baby had not been getting enough milk from me, an easy enough problem to remedy with formula top-ups, feeding regimes, relearning how to get him to latch and a medical-grade breast pump. But these practical solutions couldn't remedy what had been broken inside me. I was overwhelmed by guilt that I had let my baby down, feeling as if I was somehow 'unnatural' and failing a task for which my body had surely been designed. My loving and supportive partner, friends and family simply couldn't reach the somatic pain quietly gnawing at my insides.

We struggled on. The milk flowed and my son gained weight, but trauma caused by the breast pump and a bad latch had left me with vasospasm. My nipples were blanching as the blood vessels went into spasm, restricting blood flow. An unexpected, but thankfully not permanent, agony. But when I sought help, a different GP incredulously told me she had never heard of *that* happening before. I felt ashamed that my body and my baby were still apparently doing it wrong, but I could tell no one. Bruised but determined, we carried on. Even as breastfeeding got easier, as the pain receded and my son grew, I still carried a ball of sadness deep down, sadness that somewhere along the line we had been let down. That I let us down. Sometimes, as I nursed, I felt buoyant and full of vitality. There were many beautiful moments of pleasure. At other times, I felt like Mrs Micawber in *David Copperfield*: 'a thin and faded lady, not at all young, who was sitting in the parlour . . . with a baby at her breast.' I was disappearing and I didn't understand why.

It was at this point that I started to wonder what had happened to mothers and babies before me. I felt the itch of the researcher, that same compulsion that drove me to the edge of sanity during late-night Google searches for nipple cream or the best ways to burp a baby. One afternoon while my son napped on our bed, I found myself typing 'breast-feeding' into the Wellcome Collection's digital archive. And there in front of me appeared Victorian nipple shields. Made from wood and glass, they were thick, clumsy and crude, lacking the delicacy of modern silicone. I stared at them, shocked that breastfeeding aids were needed centuries ago, and then shocked by my own naive surprise. I dug further, through image after image, and discovered women's experiences in the fragments of their lives that remain: an ancient baby bottle found in an infant grave; a nineteenth-century pamphlet on wet-nursing; a breastfeeding sculpture from the Yoruba people of West Africa. Here was my evidence that I wasn't alone; I was now part of a historical community of parents, some of whom had also needed assistance with breastfeeding. Our circumstances and our milk were unique, but I felt bonded to this community of forebears.

Parenthood is often characterised by a forgetting, as the passage of time smooths away the sharp, painful edges, leaving frosted memories that we treasure like pebbles of sea glass. But I didn't want to forget the tug at my nipple, the crashing realisation that breastfeeding is a skill that must be acquired, or the unparalleled sense of connection with my baby. I had never experienced euphoria like it, nor had I ever felt so incapable and bewildered. If I didn't wrestle with this tumult of emotions and instincts and external noise, I'd never understand how we fitted into the bigger picture of parenthood. For every private moment when it was just him and me in our own magical world, there was me sweating and him screaming while healthcare professionals loudly discussed my nipples in front of a room full of equally bewildered new mothers. However personal our journey felt, I knew that how I fed my baby – and how I felt about it – was also a deeply social phenomenon, informed by the cultural landscape we inhabit.

It is well known that, in the UK, breastfeeding rates began to decline in the nineteenth century, falling further after the Second World War. By the 1970s, only 50 per cent of mothers were instigating breastfeeding. There has now been a swing back and rates are increasing in tandem with public health campaigns at national and international levels. This is undoubtedly cause for celebration. Yet, improving breastfeeding rates cannot depend on simply educating parents on the health benefits of breast milk and leaving them to it.[4] Because milk is about so much more. For many, breast-, chest- or body-feeding is a straightforward, painless and convenient experience. But some parents find that, far from being easy, it is a skill that needs to be learned by both parent and baby. Others find breastfeeding distressing, painful or impossible. Sometimes parents face disapproval from their own families and communities. Often, they will experience the whole spectrum of experiences, converging at one of life's more vulnerable moments. Sadly, research shows that mothers experience feelings of guilt, pressure, shame or disappointment regardless of how they fed their babies.[5]

Milk can be distressing.

Milk can also be controversial.

It is well documented that breast milk has tremendous

and unrivalled health benefits. It has economic benefits too; in 2017 the World Health Organization estimated that every $1 invested in breastfeeding generates $35 in economic returns. Yet, while we all know of the many advantages of breastfeeding, how we specifically nourish our own babies is a deeply personal, complex and emotive topic. It is about the dialogue between two beings, which begins in the first days after conception with uterine milk that nourishes the embryo until the placenta and umbilical cord take over. After birth, this dialogue is sustained through milk and it goes beyond nutrition and health outcomes, into the realms of the corporeal and emotional. For some, it is precisely this relentless physicality that means they positively decide against breastfeeding. For others, lactation is a transformative experience.

We can't talk of breastfeeding without understanding that motherhood is a social construct *as well as* a deeply felt phenomenological experience. Our choices – when we are lucky enough to be able to make them – are never made in isolation. Our options can be influenced by culture, economic circumstances, ethnicity, physiology, gender identity and more. We each carry our own unique baggage with us into parenthood, inscribed by race, class, our familial structures, histories. Our choices have always been historically dependent, influenced by societal trends and prevailing ideas of parenthood.

And what does choice even mean when decisions are never made in a vacuum? Where do choice and custom meet? Stories of universal and extended breastfeeding in pre-modern, rural communities can become myths, usually through acts of omission. For example, there is a long history of people using animal milk and other alternatives. Usually this occurred for practical reasons, but sometimes it was rooted in social custom. There are large variations across regions and time in both the numbers of children who were breastfed and the duration of their nursing. Often customs would be impacted by differences in women's participation in the labour force, as well as by rates of illegitimate births.

I found a story of a nineteenth-century woman who relocated from northern Germany to a village in Bavaria. She married and had a baby, who she planned to breastfeed, as was the custom in her homeland. Yet, in her new village it had been common since the fifteenth century to feed a baby pap – a mixture of flour, water and milk, cooked until it was thick enough that a spoon could stand upright – rather than breastfeed.[6] This was such an ingrained practice that in the village Christmas plays Mary fed Christ a meal of pap rather than breastfeed him. Undeterred, this new mother from elsewhere breastfed her baby and, in doing so, was 'openly called swinish and filthy by the local women'. Her husband was no more supportive, threatening that 'he would no longer eat anything that she prepared, if she did not give up this disgusting habit'.[7] Her decision on how to feed her baby was influenced by her own personal family history and she stood fast in the face of a community who did not see breastfeeding as 'natural' in the slightest.

Milk is always affected by social circumstances.

This book tells a story of milk through my own story as well as fragments from social and cultural history. There is a greater focus on human milk, primarily fed directly from a human body, in part because there are simply more representations of breastfeeding than other forms of infant-feeding. But there are other milks here too – from animal milk to man-made formulas – as well as other modes of delivery, such as exclusively pumping breast milk and feeding a baby via a cup or bottle. It is a book for those of us who are trying to make sense of our experiences as well as for the people who supported us. We share stories to make bonds with others, as attempts at kindness, to relieve our burdens and, possibly, to assuage our own doubts. My mother makes sense of her mothering by retelling the story of the time her daughter joined her during a night feed. Once they have left our mouths these stories morph and take on lives of their own, folded into the tales of others. Sometimes we seek them out, other times they are foisted upon us. New parents are constantly told stories because older parents cannot contain the urge to spill their own secrets, to make sense of their own journeys. Exploring infant-feeding takes us on a journey beyond a mother and baby, asking how the world sees our bodies and our communal bonds.

I am a detective sitting on a cold wooden floor, surrounded by papers and images of breastfeeding, and thinking about stories. What is it I want to remember? What do I want to know? I read once that to heal a wound you must stop touching it. But what if the cut isn't yet clean? What if grit got inside and the skin closed around it and it forever remains a hidden wound?

While researching this book, I spoke with other parents who also carry their own private and often unspoken pains. One woman told me – as so many are told – that if she tried to voice the pain of a difficult feeding experience, she was told to be grateful because her baby was now grown and healthy. All's well that ends well. But grief and trauma can haunt those who wished to nurse but found their experiences were complicated or cut short, whose feeding decisions were not respected. The wound festers silently, sometimes for decades.

Silenced when needing to speak of the lows, we are also bereft of language to talk about the highs. The pleasures of feeding babies and of bodily union and milky hormonal highs are couched in sentimentality, but also inadequately spoken of.

Words often fail us. And when they do, I have long turned to art. By exploring myths, archaeological artefacts, paintings, sculpture and social histories we can learn about those who came before us and discover ways they can help us navigate these tricky waters ourselves. Art can express the political and poetic messiness of milk. Two years after my son's last feed, I stood in a London gallery, dwarfed by a tall, wide vitrine, my eyes unexpectedly wet with tears. Encased in the glass, on a cold steel plinth at the height of my chest, was a small pink woman, her head slightly bowed. Her firm body was made of fabric the colour of pink Elastoplast, with stitching running like scars across her head, breasts, groin and knees. White threads from her nipples connected to five spools fanned out in front of her. Is she a labouring supplicant to the milk or is it nourishing her, healing her broken and bandaged body? I wasn't sure, but I viscerally understood that this sculpture by Louise Bourgeois, called *The Good Mother*, was about community and historical connections, as well as bodies that are capable of breaking and healing. The piece made me think about the contradictions of our parenthood, and how we each must recognise our own unique journeys, which are guided by the times and places of our own births. We can do this by reflecting on those who came before us. Sometimes, it is not help that we require, it is simply recognition. There may have been long nights when we felt alone, but we were also always stitched together into a vast and elaborate tapestry. Single threads can be fragile, but when woven together a textile is strong. Milk makes flesh and bone.

Part 1

THE 'GOOD' MOTHER

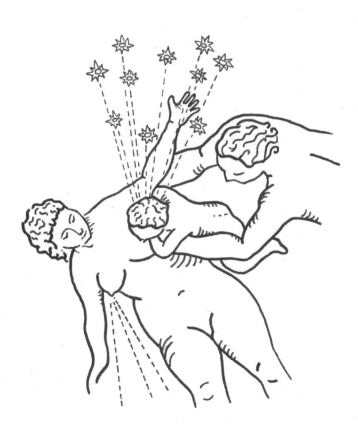

CHAPTER 1

The Magic of Milk

Carl Linnaeus could have chosen any number of defining characteristics for his taxonomy of animals but, in 1758, he defined the group humans belong to using the Latin term for breasts. The category of *Mammalia* became the sole zoological division predicated on the female reproductive organs and the foodstuffs consumed by its infants. Milk defines us. It is also our origin. Not only is our galaxy named the Milky Way, but the ultimate root of the word 'galaxy' comes from the Greek gála, which means milk. It is a fitting idea, to imagine this galactic, lactic band holding us and sustaining our lives as we float through space, each star a droplet of milk.

We see this idea depicted in the tumble of celestial bodies in *The Origin of the Milky Way*, painted by Venetian artist Jacopo Tintoretto in 1575. The work now hangs in the National Gallery in London. Against a heavenly blue background, a naked woman stumbles across a pile of lavishly decorated bed sheets tumbling towards the viewer, her left arm raised as an infant is placed under her armpit to suckle. It must have been a while since the baby last fed from her, because her let-down expels arcs of milk from each nipple. Described here, this could be a scene from the early weeks of my maternity leave: disorganised, naked and chaotic, health professionals throwing a baby at my swollen breasts. Until you notice the peacocks, the soaring figure holding the child and the cherubs that litter the canvas.

This large-scale painting is a good place to begin thinking about milk and art and bodies. Tintoretto gives us milk that is *of* a body, but which exceeds the boundary of that body. It is a work heavy with ideas about consent and ownership of one's milk and body, as well as the creative potential of milk. It is also a good place for me to begin because so much here speaks to the ideals I held about breast milk and breastfeeding. The milk here is magical stuff that flows with abandon. My mother once told me that when I was a baby, her forceful let-down had sprayed across the room. It was a story told with humour, but to me it was deeply serious. I knew that, one day, I wanted the same life force to course from my body too.

The naked woman depicted in *The Origin of the Milky Way* is Juno, wife of the unfaithful Jupiter, god of the sky. It is Jupiter, wrapped in red and blue robes, who carries his baby son, Hercules, towards Juno's breast. Jupiter had fathered the child with the mortal woman Alcmene, and needed Juno's milk so the child could obtain full immortality. But as Jupiter approached a sleeping Juno with the child, Juno woke up. (I don't imagine he was very discreet, soaring through the heavens with a hungry baby and an eagle.) And this is where we find Juno, shocked awake, one arm raised, the other pressed down into the bed, her body's openness both welcoming the child and repelling the aerial invasion. As she leaps from her bed, jets of her milk streak across the heavens. Following the trajectory of each upward jet of milk reveals that they terminate with a star, like a punctuation mark. These milky traces formed the Milky Way and mark the moment of a creation. And Hercules did manage to obtain immortality from her stolen milk.

This story from Ancient Rome originates with the Greeks. In this earlier telling, the naked woman is Hera, the often-jealous wife and sister of Zeus, the king of gods. Zeus was also an unfaithful husband and often descended to Earth to father children with mortal women. On one occasion, he tricked his way into bed with Alcmene by pretending to be her husband. The encounter resulted in the birth of Heracles. Hera could not forgive the innocent child for her husband's infidelity and tried all she could to get rid of the demigod, including sending snakes into his crib. Zeus and Hera's daughter Athena took her half-brother up to the heavens to save him. Not recognising the child, Hera took pity on him and offered him her breast. But she quickly pushed him away, perhaps because his latch caused her pain, or perhaps she suddenly realised the baby's real identity. Either way, the milk she spilled in the process created the circle of stars in the heavens.

While the painting depicts the mythical creation of the stars by a woman, its origin lies in developments in Western astronomy and the sense that the night sky and our psyche were perhaps connected. Tintoretto was close to the physician and astronomer Tommaso Rangone, a highly influential figure. The British Museum holds a bronze medal made to commemorate him. One side depicts Rangone's bearded bust, the other shows Jupiter, in the form of an eagle, holding his son to Juno's breast, who is lying naked within a band of stars. Galaxies and immortality are fitting for an astrologer-physician, whose work was concerned with extending and preserving life. As I look closely at the medal, I notice that the three stems that blossom up towards Juno are lilies.

Tintoretto may have become familiar with the story of Hercules from the *Geoponica,* a Byzantine textbook on botany that was translated into Italian and printed in

Venice in the 1540s. In that version of the story, the milk from one of Juno's breasts created the Milky Way, while the milk from her other breast fell to Earth and created the lily.

There are no flowers in the painting that now hangs in the National Gallery. But studies have revealed that it is likely missing its lower third. A seventeenth-century reproduction gives the best clue to what the missing portion might depict: a reclining nude woman with roots growing down into the earth from the fingers of her right hand, while shoots extend upwards from her left hand. She lies beside large white flowers. Is this missing woman Ops, goddess of the earth and mother of Juno and Jupiter? She was sometimes depicted nursing a baby and was associated with nurturing and fertility, so it is certainly a possibility. Lilies and galaxies made from milk.

Lilies and galaxies. I've always associated lilies with mourning, with the blankness and silence of death. But it turns out they are more precisely associated with rebirth. Does milk create life and so, logically, death too? I think about the temporal shift that took place when I knew I was pregnant, as I counted weeks, then months of my life. Doing so made death ever more real and present. The pain of labour is often described as feeling close to non-existence. Does milk's arrival afterwards signal a welcome back into light and life? The *lilium candidum* has long been associated with another mothering lodestar: the Virgin Mary. One of its common names is the madonna lily. These blooms, with their pure white petals, are often found in paintings of the Annunciation, when Mary was told she would become potent with holy life. This was the moment that Mary's motherhood was set in motion. A moment heavy with the promise of the birth of Christ. But of course, tied up in this is the story of death and, eventually, eternal life.

Milk in these stories is a powerful substance, conferring

immortality and divinity, and even creating our whole galaxy. But it is a substance that the lactating women themselves do not always control, and this is a theme that recurs again and again. Hera and Juno were the divine wives whose milk was taken from them as they slept in order to nourish their husbands' half-mortal sons. It is a moment of violence and of theft, an absence of choice and consent. Two gods fathered children, but it took goddesses' milk to make these boys divine. I look back at Tintoretto's painting, of Juno startled in her sleep, naked and stumbling forwards, her left leg caught in a tangle of bed sheets. Her raised arm makes it appear as if she is welcoming the baby into her bosom, but her blank face stares at the child in shock. Tintoretto captures the confusion of being woken and her attempt to flee from the transgression. But also, how violations against the female body are excused because they can make things of beauty – stars and lilies.

A century later, Flemish painter Peter Paul Rubens portrayed a less frenetic and more resigned depiction. Completed in 1638, *The Birth of the Milky Way* focuses attention on Juno and Hercules. Jupiter becomes a passive observer, perched behind Juno's golden carriage, his legs crossed, elbow resting on his knees, head resting on his hand. He wearily looks towards Juno and his son, as if the consequences of his philandering are becoming too effortful for him. He looks like a man who wants to be free of responsibility. Juno has spilled out of her peacock-drawn carriage bed, the red blanket falling around her legs, and the flow of her body contrasts sharply with the stiff lines and rigidity of Tintoretto's Juno. Rubens' Juno uses her fingers to cup her breast, three below and an index finger above, pressing into the tissue. Softness like this is what Rubens does best; his bodies are like butter. The jet of milk arcs downwards, behind the golden-blond curls on confused Hercules's head.

In this image it is the baby that is falling, and a question passes across his face as he looks up at Juno's. His hand reaches for the breast as his legs and body float free. According to myth, Juno pushes the baby away, but here her left hand pulls his shoulder, her fingers clawing at his fleshy arm as if to keep him upright. But her eyes look beyond the baby, into the cosmic abyss where her milk falls.

Hera and Juno's milk was divine, but the immortality it provided only held meaning within the complex web in which protagonists found themselves. This milk could only make stars and lilies because droplets fell to Earth and caught in the sky. Context is everything. Feeding is not simply one straightforward activity. It is a relationship between two (or more) people with their own preferences and needs, which change and evolve over time. Added to which, the cultural and social context is always shifting. The Earth beneath is never stable.

Our mortal milk is magic too, a creamy brew of proteins, fats, vitamins and minerals. Sophisticated and bespoke bioactive molecules help fight infection and inflammation and build up the baby's immunity. Milk production starts at roughly the midpoint of a pregnancy, the body quietly preparing itself for what will come next. In the last sweltering days of my own pregnancy, I'd lie in a cool bath for hours, running a soapy hand across the new contours of my body, curiously watching as the tiny yellow flecks on my nipples re-aquified in the water. Whatever this first milk was, it was far more viscous than I had imagined, a blooming of custard pinpricks rather than a spurt of aqueous alabaster fluids. This milk was colostrum, its golden hues hinting at its incredible nutritional and health benefits. Colostrum is easy to digest and packed full of vitamins, antibodies and proteins to welcome a baby into the world. The high concentration of white blood cells protects the baby as well as kick-starting their immune system.

This understanding of colostrum is relatively recent. Although it hasn't been universally disparaged, disparate cultures have viewed colostrum with suspicion and advised new mothers to avoid feeding their babies for two or three days after birth, until their 'proper' breast milk came in. Hmong communities in northern Thailand interpreted the yellow creaminess of colostrum to mean it was 'bad milk'.[1] Among some Hindu communities in India, it was viewed as preferable to feed the newborn cows' milk, water or honey in the days immediately after the birth.[2] In early modern Europe, physicians argued that the appearance of colostrum was the result of the excitement and heat of childbirth, which had caused the milk to curdle. It was often compared to pus due to its yellowed, viscous qualities. In 1612, French surgeon Jacques Guillemeau, best known for his work in obstetrics, described how new mothers would express their colostrum rather than feed it to their babies: 'Some women do make their keepers draw their breasts, and others draw them with glasses themselves.'[3]

I suspect that if it were produced anywhere other than from a female body, colostrum would be viewed as one of the most precious liquids on Earth, and investigated and treated as such. As it is, we have more scientific research on tomatoes than we do breast milk. A search of the most comprehensive scholarly database, Web of Science, found 10,000 scholarly articles relating to tomatoes but only 3,636 relating to breast milk; 'semen' brings up 7,851 articles and 'menstrual blood' just 239. Given the hundreds of breast-feeding images that fill our art galleries, it is remarkable that the actual make-up of breast milk only started to be fully investigated at the turn of the millennium, as evidenced by the year-on-year increase in the Web of Science search results. I shouldn't be surprised that a substance produced by women for infants was, until recently, a neglected area of scientific enquiry; milk has long been associated with other feminine secretions, which, in turn, have been considered disgusting, corrupting and taboo. It is clear, if there was ever any confusion, where female bodies have been placed in the scientific hierarchy despite, or perhaps because of, the simple fact that we have the potential to *make* life.

While the Ancient Greeks knew that human milk had metaphorical potential, they were less interested in its realities, and there has been continued ambivalence around reproduction. The creation of life is so fundamental that it hardly seems to warrant a circus of celebration. Yet it is singularly miraculous too; something is made where nothing existed, and then one must find ways to nourish and sustain this new accretion of stardust, this solid thing that now takes up space in the world. I wonder if we take the mundane miracle of breast milk for granted too because milk is always there, coded into our mammalian evolution, so that we instinctively understand, before we learn about hormones or oxytocin, that milk is related to life and to love. Yet, it is precisely because of its animalic qualities – it being of the body rather than of the mind – that breast milk has been of little interest to Western philosophical traditions.

While Hera's divine milk was the mythical creator of the Milky Way, mortal mother's milk was held in low regard. For a long time, milk was profoundly misunderstood as a substance. The fifth-century BCE philosopher Empedocles concluded that milk was pus, and Aristotle described it as menstrual blood transformed into a form of nutrition. Both views came from a belief that all bodily fluids were fundamentally the same, being variations on the theme of blood. In men, blood was transformed into sweat and semen, while in women excess blood was expelled once a month during menses, unless conception occurred, when the blood was retained to nourish the baby in the womb. Once the baby was born, this blood was redirected up from the uterus through a vein or a duct to the breasts, where it was transformed into milk to continue nourishing the baby. This idea of blood transformation endured for centuries. Leonardo da Vinci included the vein that connected the uterus to the breast in one of his anatomical drawings. Although the idea of a specifically female vein was eventually disproved, the belief that breast milk was blood remained, with the breast itself thought of as the site of the transmutation.

In early modern England, breast milk was well regarded and, because she was devoting blood to her baby, it was seen as a sign of a mother's selflessness and sacrifice. This knowledge was widely transmitted through *Aristotle's Masterpiece,* a sex manual and medical text first published in 1684 by an unnamed person or persons, using the philosopher's name perhaps for cachet. The book is full of instructions for tinctures and balms to prevent pain in the breasts, to heal the post-partum body and to help increase or decrease milk supplies as required. The book describes milk as 'nothing but the menstruous blood made white in the breasts'. This theory at least explained why menstruation usually doesn't return until a baby is weaned from the breast.

This connection between blood and milk is especially significant given the persistent idea that good health came from the balance of the four humours, a theory that originated in Ancient Greece and flourished from the medieval period onwards in western Europe. The humours, a term that derives from the Greek for 'juice', are phlegm, blood, yellow bile and black bile, all of which have a different temperature and humidity combination and play an integral role in a person's mental and physical health. The balance of humours had the potential to impact a person's emotional state as well as their physical health. The aim of the physician therefore was to achieve humoral equilibrium in a patient, and lifestyle and diet choices were recommended to maintain humoral harmony. If a patient got sick, treatments to remove any excess of one of the humours were prescribed, such as bloodletting, enemas or massage. For married couples, sex – when both parties orgasmed – was also believed to remove excess build-up of any particular humour in the sexual organs.

Breast milk was thought to be composed of all four humours, and therefore the composition of the milk was thought to influence the physical and mental characteristics of the suckling child. As the influential English physician Thomas Raynalde wrote in *The Birth of Mankind* (1598), 'affections and qualities [of the nurse] passeth forth through the milke into the child, making the child of like condition and manners'.[4] If parents were to use a wet nurse it was crucial that they selected the nurse carefully so that desirable personality traits might be transmitted via their milk. It is a belief that stretches back in time, and which can be quite comprehensive. Ancient Greek medical texts advised that a wet nurse should be Greek-speaking, so that 'the education of the child will begin in the proper language as he or she imbibes the nurse's milk'.[5] In the second century BCE the Greek physician Soranoa of Ephesus outlined the ideal qualities for a wet nurse: 'She is between 20 and 40 years of age, honest, even-tempered, pleasant, in good health, has a good complexion, is of average size; her child is less than two months old, she is clean and her milk is neither too clear nor too thick.' Writing around 900 years later, the Persian polymath Avicenna compiled a list of traits to look for in a wet nurse, who should be 'strong-necked and broad-chested [. . .] Her character and personal habits must be good, her nature equable and slowly aroused by the bad passions of the mind.'[6] He was also of the belief that a wet nurse should remain celibate, as sexual activity would sour the milk.

We therefore get a sense of how breast milk was believed to have immediate health benefits, as well as an influence in perpetuity on the personality and emotional temperament of the child. According to the famous biographer of Renaissance artists, Giorgio Vasari, Raphael was a master at painting the lactating madonna because he was fed by his own mother, rather than a wet nurse. On the other hand, Michelangelo's wet nurse was married to a stonecutter and the artist joked that this gifted him his exemplary skills: 'With my mother's milk I sucked in the hammer and chisels I use for my statues.' There are deep historical precedents that underpin this idea of relationships and bonds forged through milk. The Buddha's mother died shortly after his birth, and he was nourished by his aunt, Mahāprajāpatī. Texts emphasise that she was viewed as the Buddha's mother, primarily because she nursed him with her milk; she is often referred to as 'the Buddha's milk-mother'.[7] Her fostering of her nephew was a 'life-giving' act and, in some Buddhist cultures, a wet nurse is a symbol of supreme generosity. But bonds between nurse and infant could also be exploited. In Hindu mythology, the ogress Putana was sent to kill the infant Krishna. She gained access to the child-god by posing as his wet nurse, with the intention of poisoning the child with her milk. However, baby Krishna was too smart and instead sucked the life force from the ogress, along with all her milk.

The humoral theory anticipated what we know now from recent scientific research: breast milk is a finely tuned substance and the only foodstuff specifically and uniquely designed for human consumption. Beyond its nutritional benefits, cultures across the world view breast milk as a vital ingredient in healing medicines and to support the care of the infirm. The *Ebers* and the *Lesser Berlin* – two medical texts, written on papyrus and dating from the sixteenth century bce – recommend breast milk as a cure for many ailments, including cataracts, burns and eczema. They also give instructions for how to increase, protect and improve milk supply using fish bones, which should be warmed in oil and rubbed on the mother's back; alternatively, the woman should sit cross-legged and eat fragrant bread while rubbing her breasts with poppy plant.[8] Writing in the first century CE, the Greek botanist and physician Dioscorides included human milk in his five-volume pharmacopeia, *De Materia Medica*, which remained influential for more than a millennium. In one chapter he writes:

> The milk of a woman is extremely sweet and nutritive. Suckled it helps against gnawing of the belly and phthisis [a type of wasting disease]. It is also good to give against poisoning with sea-hare. Mixed with powdered frankincense, it is instilled in eyes that are bloody because of a blow; and applied as a cerate with hemlock, it helps those affected with gout.[9]

Sometimes, medicinal recipes called specifically for human milk. Metrodora, a Greek physician, included milk as a curative in her *On the Diseases and Cures of Women*. For inflammation she advises, 'Take the milk of a woman who has borne a male child and rose perfume. Mix together the same amount of each; heat up; take up into a pessary and apply to the mouth of the womb.'[10] The ancient Sanskrit medical text the *Suśruta Samhita*, which dates from roughly 100 BCE, credits breast milk as acting 'as a good wash in eye diseases'. Curds made with this milk are 'demulcent, sweet in digestion, tonic, pleasant, heavy, and specially beneficial to the eyes'.[11] Today, new parents are sometimes advised to use breast milk to prevent eye infections in newborn babies.

In early modern England, drinking another woman's milk was thought to speed up childbirth. Breast milk was also recommended as pain relief and was an ingredient in medicinal recipes used to treat a range of ailments from hysteria to blindness. A seventeenth-century English healer named Elizabeth Dowinge used 'a little woman's milke' mixed with herbs, honey, frankincense and urine to restore eyesight 'though near lost'.[12] Medical texts from the sixteenth and seventeenth centuries suggest that those suffering from consumption would be cured by sucking a woman's breast: 'not only for young and tender infants, but also for men and women of riper years, fallen by age or by sickness into compositions'.[13] In Massachusetts in 1752 the Reverend Ebenezer Parkman had spent the best part of the summer consumed by pain and fever and nothing had offered him comfort or cure. But by the end of August, he wrote in his diary that 'My wife tends me o'nights and supply's me with Breast-Milk.' His wife Hannah, who was at the time feeding their one-year-old child, began to breastfeed her husband too. His diary is scant on detail and so we are left to wonder if she expressed the milk or whether he nursed from her breast. In any case, within a month Parkman had made a full recovery.

The medicinal benefits of breast milk continue to be explored today. In the autumn of 2020, the Netherlands announced that approval had been granted to start collecting breast milk from donors who had tested positive for Covid-19. The milk would then be screened and administered to care home residents and other vulnerable groups as a preventative measure. Research at the Amsterdam University

Hospital had confirmed that not only can antibodies survive in milk for at least six months, they also survive the high temperatures involved in pasteurisation. In every article I read on developing breast milk as a therapeutic for treating Covid-19, I notice caveats that suggest this research is hampered by the lack of deeper understanding in wider scientific communities over the immunity benefits of breast milk. There is a sense, in this literature, of all that has been neglected and how we could be much further ahead if greater value had been placed on what some women's bodies are able to do.

It wasn't until the nineteenth century that our understanding of the infrastructure of breasts and breastfeeding increased significantly, with the publication of Sir Astley Cooper's *On the Anatomy of the Breast* in 1840.[14] Cooper was surgeon general to King George IV and later Queen Victoria, and a teacher of John Keats before the poet abandoned his medical studies in favour of the written word. Astley was also a keystone in networks of bodysnatchers, who supplied him with a constant stream of corpses, and he had a particular fascination with human breasts.[15] He explored the ligaments of the breasts, the connective tissues that hold them against the chest wall. These ligaments surround the mammary glands, a collection of ducts that converge at the nipple. Cooper used dyes and mercury to trace these networks of lactiferous tubes. The resulting diagrams look like patches of coloured lichen or trees with intricate branches reaching up and back towards the heart. But this system is far more complex than the diagrams suggest, as Cooper simplified the ducts so that they lay in straight lines. As one lactation consultant told me: men strive to make our bodies less messy.

These tissues are now known as 'Cooper's ligaments'. (So much of our bodily topography is named after the men who 'discovered' us). At the end of each duct there is a lobule, which hangs like fruit, and it is inside these that the milk is made. Cooper learned that blood is transmuted to milk in the alveoli cells within these lobules. From here, the milk travels through the ducts to the nipple, emerging from between ten and fifteen ducts like a shower spray. I recall my surprise when, swollen and ready for birth, I first tried to express milk by hand and found that the nipple didn't have just one outlet, like a garden hose; instead thick fluid appeared, as if from a sprinkler. I delighted in discovering the geographies of my own body.

On the outside of the breast, small bumps on the outer surface of the areola help the infant form a seal with their lips. Sebaceous glands within the areole secrete oils that lubricate and offer protection to the nipple. Oxytocin, the love hormone, makes the milk flow. Roughly three days after giving birth the woman's hormone levels adjust and her milk 'comes in'. Progesterone levels drop and prolactin takes over, increasing milk production. But what, precisely, is the milk?

Scientists are now undertaking groundbreaking research into the composition of breast milk. At the forefront of this research is Professor Katie Hinde, an anthropologist and neuroscientist who has conducted pioneering doctoral research into the milk of primates. Her work has contributed to our understanding of the breathtaking complexity of breast milk and the impact it has on human behaviours.

Human milk may not have formed the galaxy, but it is a living organism that contains a constellation of ingredients including proteins, fats, vitamins and microbes, the levels of which vary depending on weeks since birth, the time of day, and the needs of the baby's immune system. Milk also has its own biorhythms. Amino acids fluctuate throughout the day to help regulate the body clock. Fat content increases at midday, while the presence of melatonin increases at night to aid sleep. White blood cells and stem cells help the baby's immune system. Complex sugars, called oligosaccharides, are abundant in breast milk. These cannot be digested by the baby but are instead designed to feed the good bacteria in their tummy, preventing infection and lowering the risk of inflammation. And all of this changes to stay in tune with the baby's specific needs. When breast milk interacts with a baby's saliva, antibacterial compounds, including hydrogen peroxide, are released that control the growth of harmful bacteria such as salmonella.[16] Tasha Marks's 5318008 (2019) – to understand the title, turn the page upside down and recall being bored in a maths class – is a bronze honeycomb celebrating Bifidobacteria, one of the gut-colonising 'good bacteria' passed to babies via breast milk. The sculpture emits the smell of breast milk. In the gallery at the Wellcome Collection, I lean in closely and am surprised by its heady perfume, like Parma violets and strawberry bootlaces.

The composition of breast milk will differ depending on whether the mother has a son or a daughter, and whether this is the first baby or not. Evidence also shows that glucocorticoids – a class of steroid hormones including cortisol, the 'stress' hormone – are also transferred in milk, influencing the potential behaviour of the offspring. Hinde's research with rhesus macaques showed that younger mothers produced milk with higher levels of the stress hormone cortisol, which was associated with greater infant weight gain. But the concentration of glucocorticoids in milk was also shown to impact the temperament of the baby macaques, with higher levels leading to less confident and playful infants. Professor Hinde's research demonstrates that there exists a more complex dynamic between the mother–child unit than ever imagined and, 'just as individuals vary in their "mothering style", there is substantial variation in milk composition and yield across individuals and across time'.[17] There is still much research to be done.

Importantly, Professor Hinde doesn't fashion her research into the wonders of breast milk into a stick with which to beat women. Her obvious empathy with all species of parents is perhaps bolstered by years of watching them exhaust themselves in pursuit of nurturing. Rather than wanting to induce guilt or regret, she uses her platform to highlight the potential difficulties of breastfeeding and the need to support nursing parents, including lobbying for better economic and social policies at government level.

Sir Astley Cooper placed an emphasis on the importance of a mother's mental and physical well-being for the success of breastfeeding. According to him a 'tranquil state of mind' and a 'cheerful temper' are best for healthy lactation. He describes how grief, terror and anxiety can all disrupt milk supply, sometimes putting a stop to lactation altogether. According to him, 'fits of anger' also impact the quality of the milk, causing 'griping sensations' in the baby.[18] He recognised that there were physiological and cultural reasons that prevented a mother breastfeeding; but Cooper's list and subsequent research highlights the less-often-spoken intersection between maternal mental health and infant-feeding. Although couched in Victorian parlance, he describes what we now might understand as post-partum depression or anxiety. I recognise a modern parent who finds that feeding from their body causes mental and physical distress. But I'd never really thought to extend this empathy towards mothers who lived centuries ago; I have been guilty of forgetting that mental well-being is not a new phenomenon, even if the language and conceptual frameworks we use to talk about it now are very different.

We now know that for some, the hormonal responses to the release of milk can trigger negative feelings or unwanted thoughts. This happens when, instead of experiencing a delicious rush of oxytocin, the 'let-down' of milk causes what is known as dysphoric milk ejection reflex (DMER). Recent researchers have suggested that DMER is the result of a sudden drop in dopamine during the milk ejection reflex.[19] The result can be a short but intense period of low mood, sometimes coupled with unpleasant physical symptoms. It usually lasts a few minutes. Even less well understood is breastfeeding aversion or agitation (BAA), which can present in a variety of ways, usually as negative emotions and the urge to unlatch the baby. It is thought to be less about physiological processes and to be instead triggered by myriad social, cultural and emotional factors at different moments in a breastfeeding journey.[20] While Cooper tried to articulate these kinds of responses a century and a half ago, DMER and BAA are still not fully understood nor always accepted by medical professionals. There is still so much of milk left to explore.

It struck me, while looking at the Tintoretto as the tingle of milky fullness spread in my own breasts, that this was milk celebrated by a male painter and rendered as a sudden, very public ejaculation. The more I looked, the more disconnected from the whole thing I felt. Hera and Juno tell us of the contradictions of making milk in a confused culture. Their breast milk is so revered it is connected to the heavens, but so little was known about the milk itself.

Hera and Juno are but two figures in a long line of mothers. Motherhood has been a long-standing and persistent theme across cultures, and one particularly associated with female divinities. Often ideas overlap between cultures and times; at other times societies' views diverge. Although agnostic and a specialist of Buddhist art, I grew up in an ambient Christian society. I absorbed certain messages through school assemblies of the late 1980s and visits to see Catholic relatives, just like the society around me had absorbed similar ideas. If milk held a paradoxical place in my imagination, so did motherhood itself.

CHAPTER 2

Divine Mothers

Lived experiences and ideas about our worlds have been given material form ever since humans started carrying lamps and pigment deep into the Earth. The earliest known cave painting is in Indonesia and dates from around 45,000 years ago. It depicts a wild pig, suggesting that our Palaeolithic ancestors paid much more attention to their sustenance in their first artistic forays than they did to painting humanoid figures. If they wanted to leave their own 'portrait', they preferred to record their trace by leaving stencilled handprints. Then, roughly ten thousand years after that wild pig, the first known 'Venus' statues began to be created. These are voluptuous, faceless feminine figures made from clay and which give shape to the incarnate human experience. In the late 1980s, researchers discovered why so many of these statuettes were found in fragments; the clay had been treated so that when the figures were thrown into a fire they popped and exploded. Was this a form of ritual? Entertainment? Catharsis? Either way, from this point onwards maternal figures of people and/or goddesses proliferated.

Divine Earth mothers now run like ribbons through history. Often the Earth itself is imagined as a female body: fertile, generative and bringing forth life. This is an extraordinary power, but of a kind that has all too often been suppressed. The idea of nature itself being connected to reproduction is not an exclusively European phenomenon; it is embedded the world over, with many cultures having chthonic female deities within their origin stories. Yemoja, for example, is the primordial mother of all *orisa* (deities) found in the Yoruba pantheon. Associated with water, she makes life possible. She herself is also fluid, finding expression too in the Americas and the Caribbean, where she settled with enslaved Africans who survived the Middle Passage, adapting to her followers' needs within this complex diaspora.[1] In Haiti, she brings protection to mothers and their children. Gaia, one of the primordial Greek gods, was thought of as the very personification of Earth who sprang forth from the chaos that preceded creation. She can be found on hydrias – her torso, emerging from the ground, sometimes holding aloft an infant. It is as if she had given the soil a C-section. Thor, the Old Norse embodiment of virility and strength, was born from a woman named Jord (Jörð), whose name literally means 'Earth'.

Thinking about Earth goddesses can reveal the complexity and power inherent in the reproductive body. The mother-and-child is an enduring archetype across cultures, yet while the theme is omnipresent, it also provides a wealth of generative ideas that can be particular to specific societies. Take for example the expression of maternity found within Eastern Pende communities, located within present-day Democratic Republic of Congo. Female statues – known as *kishikishi* – are placed atop the *kibulu* (official residence) of high chiefs within these communities. These wooden finials take a variety of forms, but usually depict a woman holding a weapon. Later examples show the woman also holding an infant in her other arm, a type credited to artist Kaseya Tambwe Makumbi.[2] One striking Eastern Pende statue, now in the Detroit Institute of Arts, shows the woman breastfeeding a baby, who curls into her body.

This duality of nurturing and protection also finds expression within the Hindu pantheon. In my early pregnancy, when I was exhausted, weak and fearful, my partner returned from a work trip to Mumbai with two small statues of Durga and Kali, warrior mother goddesses whose powers of creation and destruction are celebrated as two sides of the same coin. I had studied their iconography as a graduate student. In one vivid lithograph from c.1915 Kali stands atop a male corpse, holding the head of another victim in one of her four arms as his body bleeds out beside her. She wears a garland of severed heads and a belt of human arms. Durga appears benign by contrast, riding a tiger with a weapon in each of her many hands. Although neither representation presents the female deity with a child, the inference is that the feminine can be powerful and tender, strong and vulnerable. Violent even. I placed both statues on my bedside table, as a sharp counterpoint to the helplessness I was feeling in my own expanding form.

Protection and power in the maternal form was less explicit in the imagery I had grown up with. The Virgin Mary, an Earth goddess transformed, was the divine mother who appeared at the edges of my childhood. My Irish-Liverpudlian grandmother's house was filled with her imagery and although I was raised an atheist, I found her fascinating. What a weight, to be chosen as the Mother of God! I was curious about this woman, whose motherhood fills galleries across the Western world and is centred in every primary school nativity play we attended, and so forms part of our maternal consciousness. Even when Mary is not depicted breastfeeding, in the Catholic iconography I was familiar with it is often implied. The flushed cheeks and milky skin indicate a mother dedicated to her task of motherhood. As images of Mary race through my mind like a carousel, there is one thing they all have in common: the quietly devoted 'good' mother.

Mary is one in a long line of 'good' mothers and divine breastfeeders. She emerges from a cultural milieu that includes Isis, whose agency in her own motherhood contrasts with the more passive role I felt characterised Mary's parenthood. Isis is the daughter of the Earth god and the divine mother of all the pharaohs. The ecclesiastical insistence on Mary's virginity is not present in the stories of Isis, where her determination and bravery lead to sex and conception, and thus the continuation of the power of the Egyptian pharaohs.

Isis was married to Osiris, the primaeval king of Egypt. Osiris was murdered by his jealous brother, Set, who took over the throne. Osiris's corpse was dismembered and scattered far and wide. Distraught at the death of her husband, Isis turned herself into a bird and flew across the land, collecting her husband's body and reassembling the parts into what would become the first mummy. She then reanimated her husband and in their passionate reunion they conceived a son, Horus. After this brief resurrection, Osiris descended into the underworld to become the king of the dead. As a good, protective mother, Isis tried to hide Horus from his still-homicidal uncle. She succeeded and Horus grew up, avenged his father, and fought his way to the throne.

Isis' milk was able to transfer divine powers to the pharaohs and it is believed she nursed each at their birth, their enthronement, and at their rebirth after death. Her influence eventually spread from Ancient Egypt throughout the Greco-Roman world, as far as England in the west and Afghanistan in the east. As the divine mother, Isis became the archetype for other mother goddesses throughout the Mediterranean region, including Mary.

The image of *Isis lactans* (Isis suckling) spread beyond Egypt from the eighth century BCE, on coins, amulets and small figurines. But it is not always clear whether these representations are exclusively of a divine mother or whether they can also represent mortal women. The most well-known depictions of Isis show her in a hieratic pose, seated on a throne with her breasts exposed, wearing a headdress of cow's horn. Yet other nursing statues from this period show mothers in more ordinary and familiar poses. A rare example is a painted limestone figure of a woman tandem-feeding two infants. Now in the Metropolitan Museum of Art in New York, this diminutive statue was probably found in the Tomb of Nikauinpu in Giza and dates from around 2400 BCE. A woman kneels on the ground, one knee lifted to create a hammock from her stretched skirt, which supports an infant. Both the woman and the baby hold the breast, as the baby tilts her head up to gaze playfully at her source of nourishment. Another infant crouches behind the woman and pulls the other breast down under her armpit in order to feed. The woman is wearing a hairnet, indicating she was involved in food preparation and had perhaps paused her work to feed the children.[3] It is rare for an image of a lower-class woman to be created in the round; most of these representations appear as two-dimensional paintings on tomb walls, where we find women caring for babies while they complete their daily tasks. This duality of images makes me wonder if Isis' popularity was because women of the Greco-Roman world and beyond identified with her. She gave an image to their daily, lived experiences.

In around 2500 BCE, when the name of Isis was first appearing in inscriptions in the Old Kingdom (a period between 2500–2200 BCE which is also known as the 'Age of the Pyramids') the people of the Indus region were commemorating their own ideas of mothering. This was one

of the most advanced civilisations of its time; complex
settlements extended along the Indus Valley, now in the
Sidh region of Pakistan and north-west India. This group
of cultures is now famed for its small terracotta figurines,
sometimes of animals, but mostly of women, children and
men. These have been interpreted as having a ritual function, celebrating fertility and virility. One cache of figurines,
excavated in the 1920s, contains a small terracotta figure
of a reclining woman with a baby nestled into her chest.
The baby holds a hand to the woman's breast. They are
cuddling one another. Another example, now in the National Museum of India, depicts a spherical female, wearing
a headdress and chunky necklace, the pendant of which
hangs down between her breasts, where a baby lies. It was
moulded by hand, the maker's fingers shaping breasts and
curves, pressing the mother's hands into the soft form of the
clay baby so the two hold fast together.

Perhaps this making was in itself a ritual act. Perhaps
the choice of clay as the medium connected the figurines
to the very soil of Mother Earth.[4] Life on Earth itself may
have begun in clay – or certainly the biochemicals that are
required for life came from clay, so I am told.[5] If so, these
clay models represent a cyclical logic of repetitions, coming
from the Earth and returning to it.

Isis was such an important deity that even Augustus
and Tiberius, Roman emperors with no attachment to the
Egyptian pantheon, made offerings to the *Isis lactans*. They
clearly understood that any would-be ruler of Egypt must
obtain power and protection from this mother.[6] The earliest
representations of Isis nursing show her feeding an adult
who is dressed in royal regalia. Isis, whose name means
'seat' or 'throne', bestowed kingship through her maternal protection and loving devotion. She was the ground
beneath them that enabled and supported their power.

Her breastfeeding made men powerful rulers. It was *her* power, made manifest in the act of breastfeeding, that created pharaohs. This is a quiet yet forceful kind of power, one that is often overlooked.

Mary also possesses this kind of power, yet so often her imagery has been constructed by parochial and patriarchal forces that wished to elide the potential powers of the feminine. And as societal attitudes towards women shifted, so did the way those ideals were communicated to – sometimes illiterate – women and girls through art and liturgy in the church. Representation would affect the way that communities saw motherhood and breastfeeding. In this way, the art adjusted to inexorable changes in society and, in doing so, also reinforced these changes. Thus, the image of Mary and her motherhood changed throughout time. The earth beneath us is never stable.

We see this instability of representation in just a cursory glance at Mary's trajectory over the centuries, as over time she became vitally central. In the earliest-known artistic portrayals, Mary was not associated with virginity, nor was she always depicted in the mothering poses I was familiar with. Instead, she was portrayed as a strong religious leader, arms raised, commanding attention.[7] It is during the Byzantine Empire (330–1453) that we begin to find depictions specifically of Mary's motherhood, as a mortal vehicle for the god-on-earth, after the Council of Ephesus in 431 CE officially recognised Mary as the mother of God. She sits with an infant Jesus perched on her lap looking like a little old man. The infant-as-adult is fitting for a representation that derives from Egyptian imagery of Isis, showing a king empowered from his seat in his holy mother's lap.[8]

It is only later, from roughly the seventh century onwards, that unmistakable images appear of Mary *nursing* her baby, making emphatic her role in nourishing and sustaining his human life. And in doing so, her breasts became symbolic of salvation. But this iconography only really gained traction in the West from the fourteenth century onwards. An early-fifteenth-century painting attributed to Lorenzo Monaco that once hung in Florence Cathedral points to the symbolic power of Mary's lactation. In the image, Christ and his mother are shown kneeling below God in the heavens, asking for mercy on behalf of the eight people waiting on the sidelines, each of much smaller size. Jesus gestures to his stigmata, while Mary holds her bare breast, and an inscription – a speech bubble almost – reads 'Dearest son, because of the milk that I gave you, have mercy on them.' Her breast milk was the intercessor between man and god, and a bargaining chip. It is also around this time that visual representations of the Nursing Mary became more naturalistic, the picture of the Western 'good mother' that would be relatable and recognisable to a laywoman at mass. This mode of representation peaked in the late medieval period and during the European Renaissance, meaning that today our churches and galleries are full of abundant cleavage and suckling infants. The *Madonna lactans*. The good mother.

Mary of Nazareth had, apparently, little choice in her motherhood, neither in the timing nor in the nuance of her identity or in the contours of how she would mother. It made me wonder how much I view my own motherhood through a patriarchal lens. How many of my decisions truly are my own? When does instinct get overridden by prescription? And to what extent does this complicate my understanding of my own identity as a mother?

The cultural messages I see again and again are that mothers are harassed, weary and neglected. Mothers are deeply content, happily tenacious and grounded. Mothers, including Mother Nature, are everything and nothing.

I have always been keenly aware that I *chose* to become a mother through making an active decision to try to become pregnant, something denied to so many women and girls across the world. And my choice was fulfilled – I became pregnant without experiencing the grief of baby loss, true infertility or the anguish of an unwanted pregnancy. By the time I felt ready to start a family I was in my mid-thirties and had already begun to contemplate the kind of life I might have without children. Then I met my partner and we weighed up the pros and cons until, one balmy evening in Cambodia, on the way to get a fruit shake, the conversation subtly shifted from *if* we have children to *when* we have children. We had crossed the Rubicon. I was old enough, bold enough – and naive enough – in my conviction that I could do mothering in my own way. As if I could escape the patriarchal and capitalist vortex that envelopes us all.

Acutely aware of the oppressive structures still systemic in the UK, I made a firm decision to navigate the potential derailing of my career, loss of earnings, forced redundancy, discrimination, not to mention the health risks and all the other myriad ways motherhood can disadvantage a woman in twenty-first-century Britain. According to the charity Pregnant Then Screwed, over 50,000 women (these are pre-pandemic figures) lose their jobs each year as a result of getting pregnant. Motherhood also contributes to the gender pay gap. Marginalised groups face even greater costs, and it is a scandal and source of national shame that Black people in the UK are four times more likely than white people to die during pregnancy or within six weeks of giving birth.[9]

Our choices are determined by the options available to us as individuals, and impacted by variables beyond our control. As a middle-class, white, cis woman I had the luxury of having decisions to make and there was no grey area when it came to feeding my hypothetical child: I knew I would be a breastfeeding mother before I knew for certain that I even wanted to be a mother. Before I got pregnant, I physically ached to become potent and ripe with life – in all its magic and mundane forms. In very abstract terms, I wanted to create the nourishment to grow and sustain new life. I wanted that duality of life-giving power. I imagined sitting cross-legged on the grass in the summer, holding my squishy, dumpling baby to my nipple. I watched my mum breastfeed my younger siblings. When I visited my aunt in hospital just eight hours after she gave birth to my cousin, I walked up to her bed and peeked over at the tiny baby at her breast. Within my family, breastfeeding was normalised, neither hidden nor taboo. It was talked about fondly.

Within this supportive extended family, it never occurred to me that if and when I became a parent I might have issues breastfeeding my baby. I was older and, statistically, women over the age of thirty in the UK are much more likely to breastfeed compared to younger mothers. According to the 2010 UK Infant Feeding Survey, 91 per cent of women who left full-time education after eighteen started out breastfeeding. This drops to 63 per cent for mothers who left school at sixteen or younger. Not only that, but I was also statistically less likely to come across barriers and pressures that would prevent breastfeeding. I was entitled to paid maternity leave, my partner and family would support my choices, and breastfeeding was commonplace in my neighbourhood and social circle. These are all crucial factors that feed into the likelihood of whether a parent will breastfeed and for how long.

Milk was integral to my motherhood, long before I ever became a mother. Specifically, milk produced by my body. Babies always made me think of the swell of the breast, the sweet-sour smell of my imagined child, and every Renaissance painting I had encountered as a young art history student, glimpses of smooth opaline breast tissue rising behind Jesus's head like a milky halo.

Somewhere in this cultural tangle I suspect there was the appeal of my body's potential utility as life-giving technology, rather than it being appraised like an ornament. I inhabited my body, while observing it from the outside, aware from a lifetime of stares and catcalls of how the world looked at me, objectified me, scrutinised me. Making milk made me imagine my body as something else. Maybe there was something about the logic of sex and life folding into one, into and out of my breasts.

This was a feeling that I realise is deeply personal, born from whatever combination of social, economic and cultural detritus I had absorbed and processed throughout my life. Motherhood is but one component of who I am. And milk was just one component of my motherhood. If, for me, milk was an integral part of my motherhood, then it is also true that milk extended out beyond mothering. Or beyond the confines of what, culturally, I had been told mothering was. Milk was about more than nutrition, breastfeeding more than a meal. But I didn't know any of that yet. All I knew was that I associated babies with milk and milk with my body, because this, in my mind, was what 'good mothers' did. And, when I had a baby, I would try to be a good milky mother too.

CHAPTER 3

On Birth

It was on Peckham Rye Common that an infant William Blake saw his first visions of 'a tree filled with angels, bright angelic wings bespangling every bough like stars'.[1] My experience of that expanse of grass was more mundane, but equally as transformative. At the end of the long 2018 heatwave, I hauled myself up and down the dried, yellowed grass in the hopes of speeding up the early stages of labour. I still have the selfie I took that morning, smiling with excitement and unprepared for what would come next: the raw, primal power of labouring at home that would, days later, give way to a bright, sterile operating theatre.

Just a handful of miles from the park of angels but light years away from that selfie, I found myself beyond exhausted yet still dimly aware of my desire to be a 'good mother'. For me, that meant making sure there was minimal delay in beginning breastfeeding. Milk was the beginning as I saw it, to allow us to physically reconnect after the brutality of his excavation. But our first feed was crowded and rushed. Hands on my breasts, hands on my baby's head. Groggy from the epidural, I don't remember if he latched or not after we were wheeled out of theatre. I just remember this tiny, unfamiliar being whose presence on my bare skin felt so right; but our place under the harsh fluorescent lighting was all wrong. It was as if we were in a motorway service station or an airport, those in-between places on a journey. Neither here nor there. No longer in utero, but not yet arrived at motherhood.

We spent our first night together on the recovery ward, me tentatively waddling to a bathroom that was covered in lochia, surrounded by the sounds of women, their partners and babies, and stereos. The midwives tried their absolute best to give us the attention we so needed, but there were too few of them and too many of us. At the news they'd need to keep us in for longer, I broke down, my mental health already fragile, and we were moved to a private room. Once in our own precious space, we watched the sun rise and fall from a tinted window as I nursed my son, running my fingers across the elbows, shoulders and knees that I'd already memorised from within.

Our extended hospital stay was unusual; gone are the days of confinement that were offered to my grandmothers. My paternal grandma gave birth to seven babies and was always happy for the postnatal ten-day stay in the hospital. It was the only break she ever got. That the post-partum period is delicate and requires special care is commonly understood across cultures. The ancient Sanskrit text on healing and medicine the *Suśruta Samhita* advises new mothers to avoid any physical exertion or excitement, and to stay close to their baby, as the sight, sound or touch of their infant will help lactation. Within Igbo communities in Nigeria, support for new mums comes in the form of the *omugwo*: part ritual, part practical period of time.[2] The *omugwo* usually involves the mother's mother moving in to help the household, look after the new baby, and give restorative massage to mother and child. During this time, the mother eats a specific diet to help with lactation and healing. At the end of the *omugwo* period, the new grandmother is sent home with gifts. Similar practices exist across the African continent and beyond, and point to the crucial role that community plays in motherhood – as I'll discuss in more depth later on. Women speak of the value of these long periods of nurturing and support, even as some wryly acknowledge that such a set-up isn't always without its problems.

These deep-rooted practices remind us of the importance of care and ritual in the post-partum period, which helps enable the duo to learn together how to breastfeed. It is also a liminal space and time, providing a chance for new parents and their community to adapt and adjust to changes in identity and status. A time for baby and mother to unfurl together slowly, quietly.

I know it's not helpful to compare cultures, to smooth away contextual nuances. But in that south London hospital, this was where my mind took me. In a cocoon of white sterility, we were at least able to get to know each other away from piles of washing up or the thud of our neighbour's techno. Grabbing sleep in between blood pressure checks. As I lay on the thin hospital sheets, sticky with sweat, I thought about my Cambodian friend, Virath, and his mother. One evening many years ago, just after a monsoon downpour, Virath and I were sitting on his balcony with his two young daughters, watching geckos feast on the insects that had appeared with the rains. Virath, who revelled in the quiet joys of domesticity and fatherhood, confided in me that he had never actually wanted children. This surprised me. A talented artist and natural teacher, it was as if he had been born to find contentment in family life. But he had grown up in a refugee camp just across the border in Thailand, where his family had fled in 1979 after the fall of the murderous Khmer Rouge regime that had decimated Cambodia. Virath's father had joined one of the many guerrilla factions fighting the remaining Khmer

Rouge forces in the forests across the border. It fell to a young Virath to assist the local women each time his mother gave birth. His job was to collect charcoal, which would be placed under his mother's raised bed to keep her hot in the hours and days after giving birth. I frowned when Virath told me about the fires, noticing yet again the sweat gathering in my hairline despite it being evening during the cooler, rainy season. I wondered how hot a mother needed to be in a tropical climate.

What I didn't understand then was the wider system in which this practice was embedded. That it was, ultimately, a practice of care. According to long-standing Cambodian beliefs, the body gets so 'hot' during birth it can become dangerously 'cold' afterwards.[3] It is therefore important that balance and heat are restored in the post-partum period, otherwise the woman risks ongoing sickness. Foods considered to increase the heat of the body are encouraged, as is rice wine. This practice of consuming 'hot foods' is found across Asia, including in India where new mums are recommended aubergine and dhal. The 'roasting' of the mother can take place immediately after the birth and continues for up to a week. It is also said to have the additional benefits of soothing muscular aches and forcing extended family to take care of the mother. It is a way of demarcating space and time.

In modern Cambodia, fleece often now replaces fire. Several years after my conversation with Virath, I moved to a new town and rented the upstairs, wooden storey of a house from a Cambodian family who lived in the newer, concrete rooms downstairs. As the cool season turned hot, I watched as their daughter Phally grew bigger and was eventually driven to the hospital in an air-conditioned SUV. She arrived home several days later, wrapped in thick pyjamas, a fleece and a woollen hat, which she wore for over a month.

When I asked how she was doing she smiled and shrugged and looked down at her tiny daughter at her breast. She looked weary, but happy. She was leaning into tradition, which perhaps gave her some comfort in what could be a bewildering and vulnerable time.

In my hospital room, I left my sleeping newborn and gingerly stepped into a hot shower, desperate to soothe my aching body and wash the sweat from my hair and the dried blood from my body. I tentatively rubbed my skin, peeling the tacky, blackened residue from the various things that had been taped to my skin. But I couldn't erase the bruising across my forearms and hands from each failed attempt at cannulating me, each a reminder of the many hands that touched me. In Cambodian, birth is referred to as *chlong tonle*, 'crossing the river'. That is, a time of transition, of in-betweenness, of hoping to reach the shore. The river could be choppy and the lives of those crossing at risk, or the waters calm and smooth with no unexpected currents. You just don't know until you are in the water. In Renaissance Italy, wealthy merchants would gift sets of bowls and plates to pregnant women. These would be decorated with joyful scenes of swaddled, nursing babies, allowing women to envisage optimistic outcomes for their own birth. This gave them images to help them cross the river to the other side, much needed in a time when birth was risky and plague was rife.

I remembered Phally, in her hat and fleece, and her adherence to the instruction she had been given to not shower or bathe for a week after giving birth. Not washing is a crucial part of many post-partum rituals across the globe, and I wonder if it is to preserve the smell of milk, to help the baby feed. Did my baby smell my milk in those first, confusing moments in the operating theatre? What about immediately afterwards, in the recovery ward where a tall Australian anaesthetist brought my partner a cup of instant coffee and cheerfully wished us luck, in what I now realise was a well-rehearsed routine? The baby was crying and the midwife couldn't get him to latch on to my nipple. A cannula was sticking out of my hand at an awkward angle, wires were glued to my chest. My lower body was still numb and I was afraid to hold this tiny being who didn't yet feel like mine but was definitely *of* me.

Leave us alone. Leave me alone.

I didn't want any more hands on my broken body. All I needed was someone to stoke the fires, be by our side, and allow us to find a rhythm slowly. Some newborns will crawl to the breast, find the nipple, and feed with minimal intervention. Parents have described this magical moment to me with residual wonder. But that did not happen to us. Instead, my breasts were bruised by heavy hands moulding them into a tiny mouth.

A few hours later, we were alone together for the first time, my boy and me. My partner and mum left, desperate to catch up on sleep. Despite the burning desire to be left alone immediately after giving birth, I also desperately wanted the midwife to come back and tell me what to do. Was I allowed to touch the baby? Do I need to check with someone before I feed him?

The baby snuffled and squeaked and I carefully lifted him and opened my hospital gown. I instinctively stroked his cheek and he turned to my breast, tiny mouth suckling the air, creaking and squeaking again. He latched on to my nipple, a new sensation.

And then the first clear thought I'd had in days. *I am breastfeeding. I am breastfeeding my baby. I must be a mother now.* And just for that moment, the world stopped as I marvelled at this new bodily sensation.

On a deep level, I knew my body was sustaining this strange being and that this new sense of connection gave us both continuity from womb to world. But this certainty and this sense of strength wasn't to last long, because the 'good' mother I strived to be was always accompanied by her shadow, who revealed herself to be fragile and bewildered, in need of guidance and support. What I failed to remember at that time was that there are many ways to be strong, and many kinds of power.

Part 2

THE VULNERABLE MOTHER

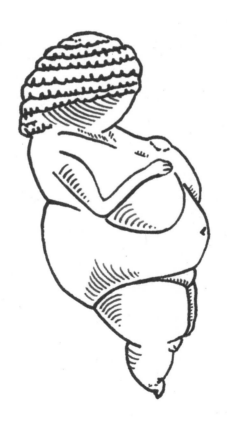

CHAPTER 4

Postnatal Bewilderment

My son is here.

From theatre, we are wheeled into the recovery ward. My gown is untied and the baby placed on my chest. I want him there desperately, so we can reacquaint ourselves through the language of skin against skin, gums against flesh, eyes searching each other's eyes. But there was no gentle reintroduction. No slow unfolding. Instead several people surrounded us, keen for him to latch on to my nipple as quickly as possible. Hands on me, hands on him, while I was silently screaming out for a moment to reclaim an iota of sovereignty over my being – and of his being, now that we were decisively divided into two beings.

I can't fault any of the healthcare workers, all of whom were overworked and overwhelmed. They wanted us to establish our mother–child connection and for my body to feed him. But immediately, a tiny bottle of formula appeared, and I don't remember if I was the one to give it to him or not. And I can't even think about it in depth because the memories of those postnatal minutes sting like a microscopic paper cut that I didn't know was hidden there, within the folds of life continuing. Was my baby's first taste the colostrum my body had worked so hard to produce, or was it the tiny sip of formula that was conjured from nowhere and given to him before I had a moment to think? Did it even matter?

Then my baby and my partner were ushered away elsewhere, so the baby could have a cannula fitted. The doctors were worried that my son and I had caught an infection during the long labour. We were to be kept in hospital so antibiotics could be administered as a precautionary measure. I was grateful to have been there in that hospital, for us to be safe and cared for, yet little of what happened, including the rationale behind the hospital's decision-making, was communicated to me with any precision.

This was already familiar to me from my antenatal appointments. From thirty-five weeks pregnant, consultants began to suggest I opt for an early induction. They had good reasons, but I needed the decision process explained to me. Instead, they wearily batted away any questions. One consultant all but patted me on the head when I came armed to the appointment, having done some research into the use of induction in my specific circumstances. In the ensuing discussion, he made it implicitly clear that he would not entertain a conversation with a *cultural historian* on such matters, even if the matter intimately concerned my body and my baby. Despite our agreeing to hold off on booking an induction for another week, I still left his office feeling humiliated and outfoxed, realising that his seemingly innocent chat about my work at the start of the examination had also been a way to find ammunition to use against me later. In the event, I went into spontaneous labour on the eve of my planned induction. After the assisted delivery and having that same doctor cheerfully explain the internal stitches he had given me while half my body was still numb, I had little spirit left. I was cowed, in more ways than one.

I felt violated and naive after the birth, annoyed by my own stupidity in not realising just how precisely devastating the process could be. A midwife gently explained how deep the bodily trauma after birth can be, late one night while I held back tears of shock at the visceral fear I felt of sitting in a position to better nurse my child because it pulled at my stitches. It left me mentally torn. Once home, I'd sit in a shallow bath and survey the foreign terrain of my body, wallowing in guilt for having left my son in the loving embrace of his auntie, his grandma, his father. I should be with him, I'd think, not abandoning him to selfishly tend to my own body's healing.

Wrapped tightly in the 'good mother' myth, I had made the mistake of thinking any concern for ourselves or time away from our baby is somehow wrong. The idea of the good mother is like a vine whose tendrils probe and squeeze every area of the psyche. To be good is to be quiet, to not complain. It is to be grateful, as if to notice – let alone worry about – the pains in our most intimate areas is a betrayal of our love for our beautiful babies. It is a woman with severe hyperemesis gravidarum who spent her pregnancy lying still in a dark room so as not to vomit again, who made repeated visits to GPs where her suffering was dismissed as her making a fuss over 'morning sickness'. Even listening to the radio made her feel nauseous, so she filled the silence with doubts about her body's abilities. It is the woman who felt pressured into agreeing to an induction, who didn't think the consultant took her questions seriously enough or gave her time to process, who felt as if she were on a conveyor belt. It is transgender and non-binary parents, who report receiving patchy support from healthcare providers, who are often ill-informed about chestfeeding, donor milk, supplementary nursing systems and pumping. It is bodies being touched without prior consent.

Where had I got the idea that my own body didn't matter? That to be a good mother was to feel full of doubt? It wasn't my family or friends, who ran hot baths and brought me home-made brownies and told me to rest. It wasn't the health visitors, who patiently checked how I was healing. It wasn't even the midwives or the doctors. It was the entire system, a perinatal journey where only my own midwife seemed to care about the sovereignty of not only my body but also my mind. Coupled with my 'good girl' inclination to look as if I was coping, to overachieve, to be doing it 'right'.

In that hour after birth, I lay in the ward feeling battered and very alone. With the 'breast is best' mantra echoing in my ears, I briefly wondered if, even though he was merely one hour old, I had already failed at being a good mother to the baby we had yet to name. But then he was returned to me, we were granted our peace, and we had that magical first feed.

The following day, high on hormones and adrenaline, like a canine ready to pounce, our new family of three made the journey to the end of the postnatal ward, where the breastfeeding counsellor was giving a talk. She spent the first fifteen minutes telling us that formula is terrible and full of things we don't want to put into our babies. I thought back to the day before, when my son was offered pre-made formula. And then I thought back to when I was eight months pregnant, sat in a windowless and stuffy hospital waiting room at our third and final antenatal class. We had covered pain relief, dilation and when to come into hospital. Now we were on to feeding.

Swollen and anticipatory, I shifted my weight in the plastic seat, my cotton maternity dress sticking to my thighs. The baby also stretched, and a foot briefly disturbed the surface of my taut belly, like a whale breaching a calm ocean. The midwife leading the session rummaged in a plastic box, pulling out a nearly perfectly spherical knitted boob.

Nervous laughter sprinkled across the room as she held a small, plastic doll to the disembodied breast, showing us the nose-to-nipple technique, which enables the baby to get the kind of good, deep latch that makes the milk flow. Satisfied that we now knew all about breastfeeding, she swiftly placed the boob and the doll back in a box and moved on to a Q&A session. A woman raised her hand and asked how best to express milk. She was at pains to point out that she planned on breastfeeding but also wanted to know if it would be possible for her husband to do an occasional feed with a bottle, if she needed to catch up on some sleep for example. The question seemed entirely reasonable. This woman was on board with breast milk but wanted some advice on different modes of delivery of said milk once her baby was a little bigger. And, given the midwife had already warned us about how tiring and all-consuming breastfeeding can be, the idea of expressing milk so the mother could rest didn't seem entirely illogical. The midwife had also already prospectively chided our partners for not taking care of us enough while we devoted ourselves to our task of breastfeeding. We knew that parents with partners who do not support breastfeeding – practically or theoretically – are less likely to continue breastfeeding beyond six weeks. The midwife could have responded by reasserting how important it can be to establish breastfeeding, or by listing the myriad other ways a partner can support their new family other than by giving the baby a bottle. Instead, the midwife shook her head and said, with a sad smile, 'We aren't allowed to talk about formula or bottle-feeding at all. We are a breastfeeding friendly hospital.'

Her avoidance of the question piqued my interest, and I was momentarily confused. I wondered why she moved on to the next question so quickly, without addressing mixed feeding – when nursing is combined with bottles of expressed milk or formula – in fact without touching at all on what we might do if bottle-feeding became a necessity or a desire. I sat there, sweaty and ripe, wondering why the options we were given were so stark, and so clearly defined as 'good' or 'bad'. But then my baby kicked again and I quickly forgot all about it. I was going to breastfeed; formula and bottles weren't going to be a feature for us anyway.

It was only much later that I consulted the UNICEF website for the Baby-Friendly Hospital Initiative (BFHI), a joint venture between UNICEF and the World Health Organization launched in the early 1990s with the aim of supporting breastfeeding globally. To gain accreditation as being 'Baby-Friendly', hospitals must adhere to a set of standards, which prohibits them from accepting offers from formula companies of free or reduced products. The Baby-Friendly Hospital Initiative has done incredible and necessary work to increase breastfeeding rates. Shortly after the initiative launched, exclusive breastfeeding rates in rural China rose from 29 per cent to 68 per cent in just two years. According to UNICEF's website, since the initiative launched in the UK breastfeeding rates have risen by 20 per cent. Yet, the ten steps that hospitals must initiate do not mention *not* discussing expressing milk or bottle-feeding. On the contrary, the BFHI UNICEF website has resources for parents who formula-feed, to help them do so safely. Their advocacy work calls for better regulation of the marketing of infant formula, so parents can make unbiased and informed choices.

During that antenatal class, our guide had confused – or conflated – Baby-Friendly with breastfeeding-friendly. And the woman who was simply curious about expressing milk was left chastened. While there are many sad stories of parents feeling shamed in antenatal classes for their curiosity around formula feeding, there are also many more who attend extremely good classes where all choices are given consideration and respect. Indeed, the breastfeeding counsellors we were to encounter later in our journey were very encouraging of me using formula, alongside supporting my deep desire to continue to nurse.

That particular exchange during our stifling class came flooding back to me the day after my son was born. In the same hospital where my baby had been given formula just hours before, I had been told about its evils. The divide between 'good' and 'bad' feeding had been reasserted and it was, seemingly, an unbridgeable gulf. But we were breastfeeding, so I forgot about the niggling sense of confusion, simmering guilt, a faint pulse of anger. Instead, sequestered away in hospital, we immersed ourselves in feeding, burping, changing, training our hands to handle this tiny being. For us, after that tiny sip of formula, breastfeeding seemed to work like a charm. The midwives in the hospital told me our latch looked good and that I nursed him like a pro. For an overachiever like me, this praise made me feel capable, unassailable. If I could perfect feeding, then maybe things would be OK. I let him stay at my breast long after his gulping diminished to gentle, sleepy sucks. I wanted him to know I was still there and that, in many ways, we were still as one. On our second night the baby fell asleep on my chest, milk drunk, and we laughed and took photos. At that moment I felt as divine as Hera creating the Milky Way. My body was making magic.

It wasn't until five days later, when we returned home in the dead of night, that I was hit by the double whammy of the weight of the physical discomfort and the heavy mantle of motherhood. And now, looking back, I can't grasp how it felt. I look at the photos, the snatches of text I wrote on my phone, but the experience itself escapes articulation. Some things are beyond grammar and syntax. It's only when I look again at one of the earliest known depictions of a female form that I recognise something of that immediate, material experience of motherhood fully realised. Here, in the solidity of stone, I find a sense of connection that expands out across thousands of years, showing me that it was possible to give shape to everything I was feeling. Turning to art was a way to remind myself that I was not alone in my confusion.

CHAPTER 5

Selfless, Faceless, Lost

The Woman of Willendorf is just 4.4 inches in height and around 25,000 years old. She is one of the best-known pieces of Palaeolithic visual culture as well as the most recognisable of the 'Venus' figures, so-called for the Roman goddess of desire and fertility. This tiny woman was excavated from the Austrian village of Willendorf in 1908. She is made from oolitic limestone and tinted with red ochre pigment, which gives her flesh a pink, textured finish. This stone is not local to Willendorf and so it is possible that she was brought there from elsewhere. Who carried her there and how? I imagine her body feeling pleasingly round and tactile in the palm of a hand; a thumb gently rubbing the contours of her hips or the coils of her hair.

To a young art history student, the Woman of Willendorf is the epitome of female sexuality and the potency and potential of motherhood. A fertility fetish. As the embodiment of sex and love, Venus was often depicted nude. The naming of these ancient naked statuettes therefore betrays early scholars' biases and assumptions about her purpose and function.

But when I look at her as a new mother, I see something else. This is exhausted fertility wrought in stone. Breasts heavy, stomach rounded, vulva swollen, it is a perfect depiction of a post-partum woman. She is faceless and with unfinished legs but exaggerated torso. In her I find an echo of my bodily experience in the weeks after my son's birth.

I want to hold the Woman of Willendorf in my hand, to feel her solidity and her weight. To me, in the early months of motherhood, she is everything, embodying both sides of fertility: the potential and the realised. She is the new mother in all her softness and depletion. The Woman of Willendorf isn't breastfeeding but is nonetheless a celebration of a woman who has likely breastfed and who will likely breast-feed again. Studies suggest that at the time she was carved, women would – if they could – breastfeed on demand, until their infants were between two and six years old. Her arms are folded over the tops of her breasts, the kind I saw in the instructional videos on YouTube that I had been shown in my local breastfeeding support cafés. These breasts are heavy and pendulous, so a baby can rest on the stomach in the so-called 'laid back' nursing position. For many this position offers an easy and comfortable way to get a deep latch, hence its alternative name of 'biological nursing'. But somehow the angles and proportions of my body weren't quite right to achieve this feeding position, and my baby didn't like being on his tummy. We persisted, yet no matter how low I sank in the rigid plastic chairs in the local library meeting room or how many times a health visitor smushed my breast tissue towards a hungry mouth, my baby and I both ended up crying in frustration. I trace my fingers over the Woman of Willendorf's image on my computer screen and feel her palpable sense of frustration too. I know the feeling travelling back through my fingers is simply my own, returning back to my heart, which is as heavy as quicksand. I have turned her into a fetish. But our connection offers me something regardless. She is also a commanding physical presence, as I become more uncoupled from my own body and more unstable day by sleep-deprived day.

Nevertheless, the part of me that needs to weave links remains nimble. I fast-forward from the Upper Palaeolithic period to today and find a thick plait of connection between the Woman of Willendorf and Louise Bourgeois, one of the great artists of our age. (Bourgeois achieved her incredible success and recognition in her later years. A solid reminder to us all to persist in the face of patriarchy.) Bourgeois is celebrated for her grappling with questions of maternity, most famously expressed through the monumental, spindly spider sculpture *Maman,* with abdomen filled with marble eggs and legs bent as if scuttling across the floor. It was she who graced Tate Modern's Turbine Hall at its opening in 2000.

But post-partum, I was not this delicate creature, spinning my web to care for and protect my babies. Perhaps that was me full of energy in late pregnancy, happily pegging white babygros on the washing line and scrubbing skirting boards. But three days after giving birth, when hormones surged and my milk came in, I was more akin to Bourgeois' *Nature Study* (2004), an ambiguous sculpture that stands at under a metre tall and which I place beside the Woman of Willendorf. The fragility of Bourgeois' white porcelain contrasts with the aggression of the canine-like creature, which sits back on all fours, three pairs of swollen breasts presented to the viewer as a potent provocation. Ribs showing, claws prominent: Bourgeois' creature is the snarling mother I wanted to be when a health visitor held my son's head with one hand and my breast with the other, pushing them together in an effort to get him to latch. Here is the unleashed animalistic ferocity that can accompany those first hormone-driven days. Here is a mother if she is allowed to express her fullness.

She has also been decapitated.

She shares this absence of a face with the Woman of Willendorf, although that is where the visual similarity ends. But I wonder if Bourgeois realised this taut canine in response to the tiny, ancient figurine. She was certainly familiar with these figures, having created her own versions of the headless women as early as 1970, first as a small bronze and later in soft textile, named Fragile Woman or Fragile Goddess. The fragility, as the artist understood it, stemmed from the fear and defensiveness of pregnancy, when an expectant parent is both afraid of their new responsibilities growing from within and afraid that someone or something from outside may cause harm to them. But what power do these tiny goddesses have beyond the potency of their own bodies? Bourgeois found a way to capture that spirit with her spider, a cultural motif characterised by irrational fears. All those scurrying legs with their thick, mottled hair. We recoil from these mothers, leaving her and her babies safe. By turning the human body wild, Bourgeois was able to depict the ferocity found in parental self-protection and vulnerability. And, except for the spider, all these works are headless.

The Woman of Willendorf has a foreshortened face with no features and Bourgeois' versions are similarly beheaded. *Nature Study* is headless, and I can only imagine its snarl. From as far back as the 1940s, Bourgeois was exploring headlessness with her 'Femme-Maison' paintings. From my bed, where I am, once again, breastfeeding, I zoom in and out of each in the series. They are simply devastating. Each nude has prominent breasts and genitalia, but all have had their heads substituted with houses. A literal imprisoning of the female subject's identities squarely in the sphere of the domestic.

*

There was a necessary rejection of the domesticity of the maternal experience by Western feminists in the 1960s, as epitomised in Betty Friedan's *The Feminine Mystique*. Published in 1963, it highlighted the oppressive effect that being a housewife and mother had on – largely white, middle-class – women. It was the important unmasking of the dark side of the 1950s suburban housewife, which Bourgeois had already rendered visible in her 'Femme-Maison' paintings more than a decade earlier.

Yet the oppressiveness of the home was not universal, as bell hooks argued in the 1980s. hooks pointed out that people of colour historically had vastly different experiences and opportunities in how they were able to maintain their family life and, therefore, rejected the characterisation of the domestic sphere as universally oppressive. She saw parenting and the associated domesticity as 'one of the few interpersonal relationships where [working-class women and/or women of colour] are affirmed and appreciated'.[1] That parenting could be empowering as well as oppressive, sometimes even simultaneously, was the crux of the feminist and poet Adrienne Rich's 1986 work, *A Woman Born*. In it, she proposed two distinct, yet at times overlapping, notions of the maternal experience: motherhood and mothering. The feminist discourse Rich contributed to was, and remains, complex: how can feminists from a pluralistic perspective 'retain the empowering or pleasurable aspects of motherhood without reinforcing the straitjacket of traditional gender arrangements'?[2] Yet it is a complexity we must grapple with if we are ever to free parenthood – including how we feed our babies – from cultures of shame and silence.

Rich defines 'motherhood' as a social construction and institution, whereby the maternal experience is shaped by patriarchy and other social conditions. This can create an often stifling and fixed identity for primary caregivers. The institution of motherhood is where we find Friedan's 1950s housewife, trapped within the home because that is where society deemed her value lay. Mothering on the other hand encompasses the sometimes pleasurable and perhaps instinctual aspects of the caregiving experience, where it can escape the confines of patriarchal institutions. Caregiving – including breastfeeding – can be a means for a woman to reconceive her subjectivity and sense of self in a way that is female-centred.[3] Mothering has the potential to be a destabilising threat to patriarchal domination, and as we shall see over the course of this book, efforts have been made to quash any true sense of maternal self. This includes the centuries-old disruption to the mother–baby nursing dyad for the benefit of male sexual desires.

Where 'motherhood' is a noun and a fixed state of being, 'mothering' is a verb focused on acts of doing. As a verb, mothering is unfixed and fluid, better able to encapsulate the multifaceted, empowering, overwhelming and fulfilling experiences of caregiving. To oversimplify it, I imagine that 'mothering' is a way of being that honours individual relationships between mother and baby, supported by an empathetic and nurturing community who instil confidence in her abilities. Motherhood is a descriptor and a definition – the state of being a mother – and in order to meet the definition certain criteria must be ticked off. A state of being where we do what we feel we 'ought' to do, where our fear of getting it wrong means we walk on tenterhooks.

Rich's distinction was a mechanism to further explore the maternal experience as it is shaped by living under a capitalist patriarchy, as well as considering moments of the experience as it can exist free from patriarchal structures. Rich writes that 'the institution of motherhood is not identical with bearing and caring for children, any more than the institution of heterosexuality is identical with intimacy and sexual love'.[4] By framing it in this way, Rich was able to draw attention to the sometimes-oppressive nature of motherhood while also allowing feminist spaces to consider women- and birth-parent-centred experiences of mothering. As Professor Andrea O'Reilly has noted, 'the reality of patriarchal motherhood, thus, must be distinguished from the possibility or potentiality of feminist mothering'.[5] Rich offers us the idea that the maternal experience can be freeing and empowering, a state of being that can offer resistance and strength, like the goddess Isis overcoming and reversing the deaths of her husband and child, enabling them to become kings. Or Bourgeois' snarling canine mother, taut power ready to pounce. But I am reminded once again that this creature is headless; any ferocity has been thwarted.

The absence of a face in the Woman of Willendorf is also jarring. We live in a culture obsessed with the face, drenched in long traditions of portraiture, compounded by the rise of the selfie. In many cultures, our face is our identity, our selfhood. But early motherhood was, for me, a time of distorted selfhood where I felt truly faceless. For the first five days of my son's life, I don't ever remember seeing or sensing my own face. And any physical sensation was entirely centred on the fullness in my breasts, the emptiness of my belly, and the bruising just below. Even when we returned home and I found time to glance in the mirror, my own face was gone, replaced by that of my son. One of my clearest memories of those days is of brushing my teeth, one hand gripping the sink in an effort to stay upright, and staring wide-eyed at my reflection, which was certainly not my own. My features had disappeared and in their place was my baby's face, his blue eyes and big squirrel cheeks. I had experienced something similar many years before, during a handful of blissful and somewhat therapeutic nights with magical mushrooms.

But back then, it was still always my face that looked back at me, albeit slightly altered. Now, leaning forward, putting all my weight onto the sink, I searched for myself while his features remained superimposed over mine. Even my face had been given over to him. It was an erasure of self.

There is an entire genre of Victorian photography known as 'hidden mother photography'. Long exposure times meant that infants had to remain still when having their photos taken, so they had to be held by their mother or perhaps a nanny or photographer's assistant. The mother was usually covered with a cloak to be disguised as a chair or hidden behind a curtain. At other times the mother was edited out afterwards, her face blackened away with only her body remaining. In some images, a blanket has been thrown over just the mother's head, leaving visible her laced clothing and a phantom arm. Sometimes the illusion works, but more often the shape of the cloaked mother is clearly visible, a ghost stalking the baby. A veiled monster pulling the luminous babies back into a void. This spectral quality is all the more haunting when a key reason parents spent money on portraits of infants was the high mortality rate.

The American artist Ash Luna has been photographing post-partum parents from across the globe for their 4th Trimester Bodies Project since 2013. The black and white photographs are celebratory and revelatory, each honouring and showcasing the variety in birthing bodies and multifaceted choices and experiences involved in birth and infant-feeding. Ash started the project with a self-portrait as they tried to make sense of the trauma of a twin pregnancy, which resulted in the loss of one baby in utero and the other spending time in a neonatal intensive-care unit. It is perhaps the most delicate of all the images from the series, and captures Ash holding their five-month-old child across their naked torso, fingers clamping their breast to help the baby latch. Their baby's head rests against an anatomical heart tattooed on Ash's forearm. But, while the tattoos point to a body that lived prior to parenthood, Ash's head has been cropped out of the image. Another erasure of self?

Looking across cultures, motherhood and particularly breastfeeding are a near-universal symbol for love. Ancient Indian texts praise breastfeeding as the sacred duty of all good mothers and compare lactating breasts to jugs of divine nectar. In Theravada Buddhist cultures, such as those found in Cambodia and Thailand, the love a mother has for her child becomes a metaphor for the lovingkindness expressed by a Buddha for the whole universe. The most obvious symbol of this love is the mother nursing her baby. And mothering, with all its compassion and connectedness, also offers an alternative path of Buddhist salvation for women who, across Theravada communities, are unable to enter the monastic orders.[6] In Thailand and Cambodia, it is not unusual for males to be ordained as a monk for a period of time – sometimes just days or weeks – in late adolescence, specifically to gain karmic merit for their parents. This is a way to pay back the debt for the care they were given as children. During the monastic preordination ceremonies, the texts recited specifically state that by becoming a monk the man can pay his mother back for her breast milk.

Breastfeeding also offers Buddhist mothers an opportunity to improve their karma. The bonds of breastfeeding are thought to increase the mother's attachment to her child, which makes future detachment more difficult. But when the time comes for her to give up her child – a son to the monkhood or a daughter to her husband's family – the mother gains karmic merit through modelling non-attachment.[7] One of the central tenets of Buddhism is that attachment is the primary source of suffering, given that everything is but temporary. Even attachment to the idea of the self is harmful. Cultivating non-attachment is paramount in Buddhist practice. By breastfeeding and mothering with an awareness of the impermanence of it all, mothers can therefore live closer to the Buddha's example of non-attachment and ultimate love.

How to encapsulate mothering in words, when it is a constantly evolving process of growth and loss and change and love? I can locate something of the essence of mothering in a photograph from when my baby was six weeks old. It was taken when two of my closest friends came to visit with their children and bottles of prosecco. I had been looking forward to an afternoon of feeling like *me* again. I curled my hair, put on make-up, and wore dungarees in an effort to look effortless. To resemble what I imagined a new mother should look like. I vaguely remember them arriving, and introducing them to my son, but I was too internally preoccupied to be present in their presence. It felt like worlds were colliding and I didn't know how to orientate myself, nor how to express my disorientation. I tried to feign breeziness, and thought I was getting away with it as two of us breastfed our babies, side by side on my sofa, sipping our drinks. It stands out as a warm, intimate moment with a woman I've known since we met in the car park of university halls, our parents unpacking matching photomontages as we eyed each other up in our velvet jackets. And here we were, a decade and a half later, mothering together, casually, as if we were still daytime drinking in our red, dingy student living room. Everything and nothing changed.

But when I look back at the photos, I don't recognise myself. There is a selfie of the three of us, holding our small babies, a toddler sitting on a lap. I shared it on social media at the time. *Look, everyone, I'm still cool!* Revisiting the photo now is near-impossible, as it evokes such an uncomfortable, uncanny reaction. On the odd occasion I scroll past it on my phone, my stomach tenses and I flinch. It reminds me that memory is fraudulent. But more than that, my evident vulnerability is painful to recall. Everyone in the photo looks like themselves: apart from me. My smile is forced and uncertain. My shoulders are hunched up round my ears and my head is pulled in and down. I look unsure, scared, shell-shocked. My hair looks ridiculous. Even my son lies on my chest at an awkward angle, uncomfortable, staring up at the ceiling, his fingers held in the devil's horns pose. The three of us, plus children, are squashed together and, although I'm in the centre, I look so removed, so very alone.

There is also a familiarity to this image; I've seen it before. I flip back down my Instagram timeline to several years earlier and find a photo taken of the three of us just after my friend had her first baby – the first of the group to become a mother. We are sat under an umbrella in her garden before the FA Cup Final, glasses of prosecco in front of us. I had just come back from Cambodia and was delighted to catch up and see my darling friend and her baby. She was so capable, so relaxed. But when I look back at this photo, she wears the same expression: hesitant, unsure, tense and tinged with vulnerability. I have never seen her look like that before or since. I put the two images side by side, peering at our faces. We were still there, lurking beneath the fogginess and the uncertain smiles. But, for a while, our faces were veiled.

This pair of photos punctures me. What the camera captured was not what I had prepared and posed for. Instead, both these images record an in-between moment in a longer period of change, between what we were before and what we were becoming. This was a moment where we were figuring out how to grow and find power in this change. By birth, by motherhood, by giving up our bodies again and again. Something we could do side by side, but also, ultimately, alone. But I was never supposed to see this so clearly from the outside.

Aside from the pervasive idea of the Woman of Willendorf as a fertility fetish, a mother goddess or similar, there is another theory that she is actually a self-portrait.[8] For me, this idea holds weight. In the 1990s, anthropologists Catherine McCoid and LeRoy McDermott had photographs taken from the perspectives of women looking down at their own bodies, in the same manner as this ancient statue. When placed next to corresponding views of the Woman of Willendorf, the similarity is striking. Practically speaking, the foreshortening of the leg and the stoop of the face is what a body looks like when appraised by its inhabitant from above. Whoever carved this perhaps used their own body as a reference. Maybe it was made by a woman who remembered what it felt like to be faceless too, the loss of herself driving her to realise the transmutation of her form, of her being. To look at herself anew and to sculpt it from the outside. Giving shape in clay to make sense of the bodily sensations, the numbness, the rawness. Maybe she wanted to say: *Here I am now. I am still here.*

Meanwhile, I was still lost. The amorphous idea of the 'good' mother stalked my post-partum months and, like a faulty compass, ensured that I never quite felt as if I was on the correct path. Was I wrong to leave my partner to soothe our newborn while I took a quick shower? Should I feel guilty, despite the fact I was so full of drugs and exhaustion by the time I finally met my son, that it had taken a while for that rush of recognition? How could I keep getting breastfeeding so wrong? When an older lady admonished me for not wrapping him up sufficiently, during an unseasonably warm September in an overheated shop, I fought back the tears and doubted all my instincts. I knew I was right, but still I wondered whether I was not devoted enough.

Now I can see how in those early weeks, the parenting tasks are distilled down to simple survival: feeding, sleeping, cleaning, protecting them from harm. So many emotions coalesce around feeding our babies because, in those first days and weeks, it is one of the only things we must do. It is the central task.

I knew, on a deep level, that ambivalence, guilt, annoyance, uncertainty were all entirely normal feelings. But it was hard to maintain any fortitude in the face of the deluge of uncertainty and the weight of being chosen as this precious infant's mother. I thought back to all those divine mothers, but I couldn't ride a tiger or fuse with the Earth. My milk didn't flow with abundance, nor did jets of it arc across space. Still, I nearly always felt the burn of a hundred eyes on me, scrutinising me like an art historian studies painted surfaces. Most of the time these stares were figments of my imagination. Yet seeking support with breastfeeding meant that at least once a week I became the object of enquiry through the evaluating eyes of health visitors, breastfeeding counsellors and other well-meaning helpers. I felt lucky to have this support but, without a stable sense of self, it often left me feeling further fragmented and unsure of my own agency.

The ultimate Christian symbol of motherhood is generally not a woman in possession of agency over her divinity. Her motherhood is also the subject of scrutiny. Rogier van der Weyden's *St Luke Drawing the Virgin* (1435–40) is an apt illustration of the bind that Mary found herself in. Depictions of St Luke drawing Mary from life are abundant. Some of these were believed by the faithful to have been painted by St Luke himself, after Mary came to him in a vision to enable him to produce a true portrait in her likeness. In many versions, the saint is seated at an easel capturing the posed Mary gesturing to her son. She is aware of her own objectification. But in van der Weyden's painting, it isn't clear Mary knows she is being watched. To the left of the scene, she sits on the steps of a throne, lavishly dressed, expertly 'sandwiching' her breast tissue with two fingers shaped into a V so the nipple will angle into Jesus' mouth for a deep latch. After the careful cleaning and restoration of the work in 2015, a painted drop of milk was found. Mary the milk-giver. She gazes down at her son, lost in an act of feeding, a moment perhaps of warmth, bonding and mothering. But then, just across the pictorial field, we find St Luke, kneeling with an inconspicuous sketchpad in one hand and a poised stylus in the other, appraising Mary's motherhood.

St Luke's presence is a metaphor for the way the mothering experience can turn to Adrienne Rich's motherhood by being monitored, scrutinised and adjudged. Judgement – perceived or imagined – is ingrained in our cultural attitudes towards parents. Mary appears uneasy under the saint's gaze; her body is angled and stiff, she cannot relax. Even the baby is rigid. There is none of the recalcitrant, fleshy voluptuousness associated with feeding an older baby, which Jesus evidently is in this image. Where is the chubby hand exploring his mother's mouth or grabbing fistfuls of her hair? How I identify with Mary's posing! How many times did I assume the posture of a composed, unflappable mother while in public? How many times did that composure fall to pieces within the privacy of my own home, when my partner would find me crouched and sobbing on the nursery floor? Mothering? I could do the mothering, but the weight of feeling as if one's motherhood is being constantly observed and judged? That's a mantle that can wear you down.

Until I looked back at that photograph of me and my closest friends, I couldn't see how vulnerable I looked from the outside, nor did I know how to make these fears understood by others. The core of my identity – even my recognition of my own face – had melted away. Beneath the carapace of clothing and slicks of red lipstick, I was a walking wound.

CHAPTER 6

Leaking Bodies and Let-Downs

Let me take you back to 2017. I am beside another of Louise Bourgeois' spiders, which dominates the gallery space in the newly opened wing at Tate Modern. She is magnificent. But on that day, I was transfixed by a grid of sixteen of the artist's mixed-media works on paper, filling the wall facing the arachnid. The series is called *À L'Infini* (2008–2009) and each drawing is a tangle of tubes that snake across the wall, diverging and wrapping round one another like an umbilical cord. Some tubes terminate with sacs containing floating astronaut babies, others end with globules of cells. Watery female bodies get twisted in the knots. Everything is in shades of red gouache, which bleed out across the white pages. Bourgeois frequently worked in red. Red for blood, red for anger. In another series, she repeats the motif of headless, limbless pregnant bodies with stick babies floating in the womb cavity. Elsewhere, babies fly from bodies with cartoon heads or multiple breasts hanging like grapes. She's humorous, this artist. Philosophical, but funny.

But I couldn't feel the amusement in 2017. My body desperately wanted a baby and a gnawing hollowness in my abdomen made itself known to me. I also knew I was running out of time. Red for an alarm. I had a basic sense of what welcoming a baby into my life might involve. And in that imagining, I assumed I would breastfeed and that, in the whole process, my body would change. At the time, I didn't understand that I might feel exactly like that faceless female body, barely tethered, edges bleeding out into white void.

A year later, these visceral, red images came back to me. I was in the first months of my pregnancy and my body was in a constant state of flux. The baby was an abstraction. A pregnancy test had confirmed it was there, but the only proof of life came from the hyperemesis that had me hunched over a toilet bowl multiple times a day. Vomiting was one of many disparate symptoms of an invisible presence. Slumped on white tile, I pictured a stick baby roiling in my stomach, pushing at my ribs, excavating space for themselves. I held my breath and kept my silence.

Eventually, those symptoms passed. Once that happened, my mind began to calm, and my baby stretched my belly out to an ultimately unbelievable size. I loved my body in those months, as it vividly yet gently spun my baby closer to existence and he made his presence known through somersaults and kicks. My body was now very clearly somebody else's home and I had developed an intense, protective love for the stranger who inhabited me. My body was a house and I felt perhaps more at home than at any other time of my life. I was fecund and rounded and *contained*.

Until, early one August morning, I was no longer contained. Suddenly everything was on the outside, going out beyond the borders of my body and into the world. Immediately, my body became an unstable and unsightly vessel.

First and most obviously was my baby, but that was OK. He was an acceptable evacuation, squishy and small and otherworldly beautiful. But then came the lochia – the bloody, heavy discharge, sometimes accompanied by small clots, that can last for weeks as the womb sheds and replaces its lining. This was accompanied by the sweats, as hormone levels changed and my body released excess fluids. Lastly, three days after giving birth, my milk came in.

Leaky. Floppy. Squishy. Stretched. Saggy. Deflated. The abject body, as Julia Kristeva would say. That is, in all its oozing and messiness, my body was repulsive and grotesque. She writes, 'It is thus not lack of cleanliness or health that causes abjection but what disturbs identity, system, order. What does not respect borders, positions, rules. The in-between, the ambiguous, the composite.'[1] It is not so much the perceived uncleanliness of the leaking milk or vaginal blood that causes offence, but instead the way this disrupts and exceeds the borders of the body.

While my stomach slowly deflated, my breasts cycled through swelling and slackening. Beneath my clothes, as my vulva healed, my nipples became pinched and raw. These are the silent places, the places that a woman must never refer to, the places my culture does not really want to think about, outside of sex and seduction. Instead, I was aware that my body should be silenced and that I should conceal any evidence of my normal, functioning *post-partum* body. I was to pad myself, cover myself and pretend that nothing was happening. Mostly, I was to construct and respect the borders between body and the outside world.

There was no template for how I might begin to bask in my body's gory glory. But there were rare occasions when I managed it. And, when this happened, it was focused on milk – the most acceptable leakage. When my son slept through a night feed and I would wake with soaked bed sheets and concrete breasts, allowing myself to pause just for a minute in the dampness, luxuriating in my body's abundance. Because for much of the breastfeeding journey

I was afraid my body was not enough, and now here was the proof that it was being productive. (I was still labouring under the idea that my body had to be of use and needed to have some value to be worth celebrating.) But I could never luxuriate in milky abundance publicly. Is it the softness of the breastfeeding body that is so animalistic and, therefore, potentially offensive? Was it that my body was overflowing with *stuff*, the type that Western culture viewed as disgusting? Disgust, a basic emotion, designed to protect us from pathogens, can also be elicited by socially shaped transgressions. Bodily fluids – particularly those from the female body – become viewed as potential contagions.

Red for danger. White for purity and newness. But for much of Western history, breast milk was believed to be menstrual blood transformed. Disguised. Disgusting? The parallels between breast milk and menstrual blood persist. Both are bodily fluids that are associated with the sexual organs of the female body, so it is unsurprising that revulsion and taboo surrounding menstrual blood can be transferred to milk. The equivalence between these bodily fluids has had an impact not only on how breastfeeding is viewed by society, but also on how women themselves think about lactation. Noting the inadequacy of public health campaigns that simply inform women that breastfeeding is best, Professor Ros Bramwell suggests that the way we internalise societal ideas about our bodies can impact how we choose to feed our babies. In a preliminary study, she tested the idea that attitudes towards menstrual blood can influence a woman's views of her own breast milk. The results showed 'significant relationships between some menstrual attitudes and attitudes to breastfeeding'.[2] Her research of women and men in the UK indicated that positive attitudes towards menstruation correlated with positive attitudes towards breastfeeding. Conversely, those who felt menstruation was 'bothersome' were less likely to report positive attitudes to breastfeeding. We are not born with these attitudes. We internalise them, years of shame settling into our cells. How can we simply tell a woman that her breast milk is best, after she has endured a lifetime of being told her body is – somehow – shameful?

For all the beautiful images of breastfeeding conjured in words and pictures, it remains true that the lactating body has long been deemed inferior to the male body. The Christian lactating body could be holy, but it was also a consequence of Eve's fall and expulsion from Eden, part of a package of suffering to be endured by all women for the so-called crime of seeking wisdom. Plato saw the body as vulgar and deemed women's bodies to be particularly disorderly. This is also true in Buddhism, where woman-hood is an inferior state compared to being born as a man. We are 'corrupted beings', in part due to our attachment to sensuous desires in previous lives, incarnated within a body that can pollute and contaminate. While this example comes from a broad gloss of Buddhist thinking, it speaks to the way the maternal experience is always bisected into these contradictory bodies: the maternal body, full of love and milky potential, but a body that is also corrupted and, perhaps, corrupting.

When my son was twenty-eight days old, a midwife came to our flat for her final visit. She sat with us for nearly an hour, helping me to breastfeed. She helped position me within a fort of supportive cushions and was the first person to show me how to look at the movement in my baby's ears and jaw. When his ears wiggled it meant he was swallowing, whereas the small, flicking movements like butterflies against my nipple indicated he'd finished feeding and was enjoying the comfort my body offered him. I was beyond grateful for her time and her gentle presence and encouragement. At the end of the visit she weighed my son with the old-fashioned hanging spring scales. My naked fish baby. My catch of the day. She handed him back to me so she could plot his weight on his chart, and quietly did some calculations. But I could already see with my eyes and feel with my heart that he had lost too much weight. As it was a weekend, the midwife told us to go to A&E.

Waiting in the consulting room, I felt both betrayed and the betrayer. Stricken, I felt as if I were disintegrating as I sat on another hard plastic chair, my son wrapped against my body in a soft cotton sling. We were seen quickly and they tested for all kinds of problems that could result in weight loss, such as issues with his thyroid. But it quickly became clear that the problem was with breastfeeding.

I mentally translated this as being a problem with me. A problem that was entirely my fault. Distraught and guilty, I couldn't help thinking it was all thanks to my somehow deficit body. (What a cruel and unforgiving appellation, especially for a body that has never failed me and which had just grown and birthed a new human.) Still, a glimmer of resentment flickered inside me, for being in hospital and not curled up in bed at home. Instead, I perched on a fold-out bed, reading the ingredients on a tiny plastic bottle of pre-prepared formula. This time I was definitely the one to give it to my son, because I clearly remember a voice in my head repeating words I had read somewhere, once long ago: formula is akin to poison.

Even back then, when I read those words, I never believed formula to be anything like poison. It is true that studies often find correlations between breastfed babies and better outcomes. Yet, for ethical reasons, these studies tend to be less able to account for confounding variables; it is impossible to isolate feeding from other lifestyle and health factors, which may also impact health outcomes. Some of the kindest and cleverest people I know were fed on formula and I know many incredible parents who, for a variety of reasons, fed their own healthy babies with formula.

That said, I did not consider formula to have a place in the motherhood I had envisaged for myself – an ideal I had conjured from all the cultural and societal references I'd absorbed over my lifetime. This unique combination of factors shaped my vision for how my motherhood was to be. But I also desperately wanted my body to continue making life, to make the substance that connected me to him. For me the struggle with accepting formula was not only the quantitative differences in terms of nutrition and composition, but the removal of my body as an essential component in feeding my baby. I wanted to maintain that physical umbilical cord. I wasn't ready to let go.

It is difficult to find the language and cultural references for all of this. We have the Ancient Greeks to thank for the contradictory values placed on maternal work and breast milk, given how much they downplayed the generative contribution of the woman in reproduction. Plato was clear on this: men 'sow upon the womb, as in a field, animals unseen by reason of their smallness and without form'.[3] Aristotle qualified this by making it clear that conception was the result of the male seed only. Female bodies are the inert hosts; it is the sperm that is the animating force that sets creation in motion. Men are active; women merely provide the receptacle. We see this continue as Christianity places emphasis on the spiritual and metaphorical aspects of motherhood, while 'the physical aspects of motherhood were increasingly left in the shadows and laden with negative connotations, as something animalistic or shameful; childbirth was surrounded by the taint of impurity'.[4]

All of which, of course, ignores the expansiveness of

pregnancy, birth and lactation. A woman from the east coast of the USA told me that breastfeeding in the early days made her feel as if 'my brain was just growing, like when learning a new language by immersion'. Another told me breastfeeding softened what felt to her like the brutal separation that occurred between her and her baby during a birth by C-section. She described breastfeeding as a slow recoupling. Another woman, who had been very ambivalent about breastfeeding before she gave birth, said nursing her small baby 'felt as if I was still making her'. Breast milk is generative; it is a daily act of creation.

For those who wish to breastfeed, being unable to do so can be wounding. The tiny bottle of formula was a symbol of the failure I perceived in myself. Worse was that my body had tricked me into thinking it was doing its job, when really my little boy hadn't been getting enough milk. I threw the bottle into the bin and looked over at his little body tucked into the blanket nest a nurse had made on the bed. I tried to sit on the metal pipes that ran along the wall, texting my best friend to tell her we were in hospital. I wrote a long, rambling message that could probably be distilled down to: *My baby was hungry and I didn't notice. I failed to make him milk. I have failed as a mother.*

Shortly after pressing send on this sad little missive, a nurse appeared to explain how we should 'top up' my son with a precise amount of formula, while our feeds should be evenly spaced every three hours and precisely timed. Suddenly, we were in a world where breast milk and formula were coexisting and no one was refusing to talk about bottle-feeding or deriding formula as poison. Everything I had been told before felt oversimplified. All I knew was that I wanted to breastfeed, I wanted him to drink *my* milk, but, in that hospital, I felt as if I was ultimately being pushed to abandon breast milk altogether. This was compounded by being told, initially, that I should do a full feed from both breasts, then give a formula top-up, while pumping. This in itself took the full three hours between feeds. It was only the following morning that the error was noticed, and I was advised to only nurse for ten minutes. As soon as the doctors confirmed that our issue was with feeding, we asked to see one of the hospital's lactation consultants. She arrived just as we were being discharged. She did not want to watch us nurse. She looked down at my son, still sleeping in a bundle of blankets on the hospital bed, and told us she was used to working with newborns and so couldn't help my four-week-old baby. She told us to see someone privately.

I am aware of how ungrateful I sound, talking about life and betrayal when we were on a ward with truly sick children, whose cure wasn't as simple as a bottle of milk. I know that for some parents, the ritual and routine of expressing milk can provide a rhythm that allows them to negotiate the distress and unknowns of having a baby in a neonatal intensive care unit. Though I felt broken, I was still aware that I possessed a deck of cards stacked in my favour. I never had to carry the additional weight of wondering if – or knowing that – the care I received was influenced by the colour of my skin, the accent in my voice, the name on my notes, or my gender presentation. Yet at the time, I was mired in solipsistic new motherhood, sleep-deprived and myopically focused on my baby and little else. All that mattered was us. Keeping him alive, proving to myself that I was capable of the task. I wasn't Renoir or St Luke with their paintbrushes, observing the scene from the outside. I wasn't even my partner, who could walk out of the house at 8 a.m. and not return for a whole eight hours. I was tethered, just as Louise Bourgeois knew, with her babies still attached and floating around the woman, as if on an extended umbilical cord. And because milk was so integral to the whole damned enterprise for me, I was preoccupied with the precise kinds of milk I was nourishing him with.

Many women in the UK experience something similar. According to 2010 figures compiled by UNICEF, 81 per cent of birth parents in England initiated breastfeeding at birth. However, by the time the baby was six weeks old, the number of parents exclusively breastfeeding had dropped to 24 per cent. By 2019, breastfeeding rates at six to eight weeks had risen to 48 per cent. While this data also includes babies who were not exclusively breastfed, it still points to improvement. Yet rates in the UK are still comparatively low and still plummet within a few weeks of birth. For the majority of these parents, the decision to clip closed the nursing bra is not made easily. Professor Amy Brown's research demonstrates that 90 per cent of women who stopped breastfeeding by six weeks were not ready to do so, for reasons often linked to lack of support, a sense of social stigma, negative reactions from loved ones, inconsistent advice or complications. This can leave many parents with complex emotions, from frustration to feelings of grief.[5] I was not alone in mourning every lost feed with my son or fearing the loss of the relationship I had hoped to have with him.

We walked out of the hospital, my son wrapped against my chest, with instructions to feed from both breasts, then give him a bottle while I connected myself to an industrial pump to try to extract the next top-up from my exhausted body. For the next week I followed this routine religiously. Nurse, top up, express, sterilise, cry. Every three hours. We set alarms, meticulously timed feeds and tracked my output by the millilitre. As I gratefully and resentfully measured out spoonfuls of powdered formula, questions of nourishment consumed me. I was confused, navigating this hybrid world of breastfeeding and formula, with no familial precedent to guide me and no way of understanding how this fitted into an ideal of breastfeeding as a 'natural', timeless activity. No one had told us when to stop this tortuous regime. No one told us that this is mixed feeding and that it can happen all the time. No one said that formula feeding and expressing didn't have to mean the end of breastfeeding, but that they could all coexist. While my bed had become an intensive dairy farm, not one solitary healthcare professional or lactation consultant gave us husbandry guidance for this new equipment. I knew nothing of flange sizes, or how to mimic the rhythms of the baby's suctions to draw out the milk. Despite being a researcher, I simply lacked the energy or will to read about how to properly pump. I look back now, baffled that we didn't consider a more expensive breast pump to be a worthy investment – that the correct equipment for me was so low on our priority list.

We were passed from health visitor to GP to peer supporter. No one seemed to know what to do with us or with my quest to continue breastfeeding. My GP didn't understand why I wanted to continue despite the physical pain, despite the thrush in my breasts that no one believed me about; I can't even tell you the problems we had treating that. But I can tell you about the weeks of deep, lingering pain. The agony. Of biting down on my knuckles and the fear of the next feed. I remember reading somewhere: 'don't tense up otherwise the milk won't let down.'

When I was clear I wanted to continue breastfeeding but needed help to manage the crippling pain it was causing me, the overriding message I got given was that I should just be grateful to be breastfeeding. As if being able to bask in their praise was enough to help me hold my tongue when it came to my own bodily complaints. Deep pain in my breast tissue? Feed through it. No blood supply to my nipples, causing excruciating pain and fear? That simply doesn't happen, so you must be wrong. I thought of all those Madonna and Child images, I thought of Renoir's wholesome wife, the way paint glosses over women's bodily experiences, their traumas and pains. Their mental anguish and emotional turmoil.

'Mummy, hey, Mummy! You feel them sucking the life out of you, don't you?' My eyes remained focused on the sunlit patch of grass I'd been staring at. The question couldn't have been aimed at me. A moment of quiet had allowed my mind to wander and it took me a beat to realise the woman at the far end of the bus stop was talking to me. How did she know I was a mummy? Oh yes, the pram containing a baby. He was six weeks old and, somehow, I'd summoned the energy to dress properly for this trip to register his birth. Long black dress, dark red lipstick, hair washed and styled. Each step getting us from bedroom to registry office offered a momentary escape from the constant preoccupation with my son's weight gain, with the number of millilitres of milk I was expressing, the volume of breast milk stored in the fridge, the number of formula top-ups I would allow at bed-time, the niggling arguments about night feeds and nipple confusion.

I turned to smile at this woman who had addressed me, noticing her overstuffed shopping trolley, in which I could see an old VHS machine. 'It's hard isn't it,' she said, more of a statement than a question. I smiled and gave a polite nod. There was an old man sat between us and I didn't want to subject him to the messiness – literal and metaphorical – of new motherhood. But she persisted, uninhibited, and asked again, 'You know when they are feeding and you feel the pull, like the life being sucked from you?' I couldn't summon any words, and simply nodded again.

I thought I knew what she meant; thought she was

referring to the physical sensation. It was only later that I understood the full weight of her words, and I still sometimes silently thank her for her sympathetic intrusion.

Because I was being depleted. Each feeding challenge felt like a wound; to my sense of who I wanted to be as a mother, to my expectations. I believed this was something I had to endure, a test of mettle that would determine who I would be as a mother and as a person. My partner tiptoed around the issue of giving up breastfeeding; our conversations were like minefields. I was fortunate that he continued to support my dogged persistence. Each day, he would trek out to buy the latest requirement: breast pumps, nipple shields, food to help my milk supply. I could see his concern and love. He watched me sobbing. He watched me in agony and begged me to let him make up a bottle of formula. Sometimes I relented and each time I was overcome with sadness, which came from a place he simply couldn't understand, despite his best efforts. He didn't see that, to me, each bottle was a tiny grief. Even the smell of formula was wrong; it made my son smell different. My struggle was twofold and at times contradictory. There were days when the relief from the burden of it all was overwhelming. Yet mostly I watched with jealousy as my partner fed my son his night-time top-up feed. I felt betrayed because at the time I understood that what was being 'topped-up' was my body, which had been unreliable and untrustworthy.

Once again, I was forgetting myself and falling into the milky myths that muddy breastfeeding histories, that smooth away the fact that motherhood and childhood are social and cultural constructions. You are probably familiar with these stories. That women in this part of the world all breastfeed happily until a child is three years old. Women in that part of the world breastfeed without any problems at all. These are stories boiled down to their essence, then applied to whole groups, any group that is somehow 'other' to our own. One such emblem, which I encountered numerous times during my research, is the idea of a breastfeeding Utopia. I most frequently encounter these on breastfeeding blogs written by women who are noble in their aims to promote breastfeeding, if a little lacking in nuance. Sometimes, the Utopia is an idyllic time in a vague past, before the incursion of modernity and medicine. At other times, it is an othered and exoticised location, often imprecise in its geographical scope and regional specificity. 'Africa', for example. These stories omit the fact that, for all the trust we *should* place on our miraculous bodies, we are still bodies existing within a whole vortex of influences. These milky myths are just fragments of breastfeeding know-how or information, which have been distilled down even further and fashioned into totems of breastfeeding lore. When employed as a point of comparison for my own experiences, all they ever really did was shame me. They made me feel diminished.

Mongolia is one such talisman and it is worth unpicking this example in more detail. It is true that Mongolia has an extraordinarily supportive breastfeeding culture. Yet the complexity of it has transformed, in contemporary breastfeeding blogs, into sweeping general references to Mongolian women and cups of left-over breast milk, with no sense of context. While there are undoubtedly better times and places for supportive breastfeeding practices, what these fragments often omit are how different social and cultural norms are between Mongolia and western Europe or North America. I can see how these ideas can feel like a balm to a breastfeeding mother in the West when, confused about why, if breast is best, she has also been forewarned about potential problems if she tries nursing in public. Stories like this can be useful when a relative quietly 'suggests' feeding the baby upstairs, lest the male adults in the room feel uncomfortable. Stories of *something* or *somewhere* where breastfeeding is more readily accepted are a rock to cling to when smuggling a breast pump into work, shuffling off to express in the toilets so as not to cause fuss or offence. Being able to evoke examples of places where breastfeeding is wholly accepted and commonplace – and not taboo – helps conceive of a world where women could be better supported, even if those examples are inexact. This can be better.

As with all good myths, there is truth in them, but as the story becomes distilled, so the specificity of the context gets smoothed away. The cultural and social differences between, say, London and Ulaanbaatar are vast, not to mention the differences between suburban UK and the Mongolian steppes. It is in the granular detail where these idylls become less useful. By not acknowledging the cultural differences that impact upon parents and their child-rearing choices, mythical places where breastfeeding is always supported become not only sticks with which to beat back oppression, but also sticks that can be used to beat ourselves. How many times did I ruminate over these mothers elsewhere, without factoring in the vast differences in community support, best practices, localised knowledge and more?

I speak with Professor Rebecca Empson, an anthropologist and mother who has spent over twenty years working in and on Mongolia, primarily researching women and economic development. She agrees the culture in Mongolia is much more breastfeeding-friendly than in the UK, but that this can be explained by the broader cultural context in which breast milk belongs. And, over the course of two decades, she has witnessed changes in infant-feeding practices, tied to social and economic changes.

Mongolia has a much stronger 'milk culture' than other

places. Writing on the place of milk in rural Mongolian communities, Dr Ariell Ahearn, a specialist in Mongolian culture and social relations, points to the specific context in which milk belongs, arguing that it plays an integral part in community and social bonds. She spent long periods with women as they milked their animals. This milk is a central part of life in rural households.[6] Milk also forms an important aspect of ritual and religious practices, some of which are practised daily and usually by women. This has a long history: contemporary accounts of the life of Genghis Khan, the founder of the Mongolian Empire, record him ritually sprinkling milk, and Marco Polo notes milk libations in his accounts.[7] There is greater presence of milk, as well as closer proximity to the rhythms of milking animals. And, until relatively recently, there were no real alternatives to breastfeeding, with little formula and few bottles on the market during the socialist period. In addition, remote communities had no running water or electricity, and so if a woman couldn't produce milk then their only options were to have their baby fed by another woman or mix cows' milk into a pap-like substance.

Generally, breasts were not fetishised and, consequently, there was less demarcation between self and identity, both before and after motherhood. And, as in many places, the community tends to be highly supportive of new mothers in the post-partum period, and breast milk features heavily in this care. If a mother's milk supply is disrupted it tends to be attributed to the mother not being given sufficient attention or gifts in the first days after the birth. Milk becomes the tangible result of nurturing and care.[8] This belief is functional and ensures adequate support in the first weeks of parenthood, ensuring the mother doesn't get sidelined completely when the new baby arrives. (I have heard horror stories of new parents in the UK being expected to make tea, and sometimes entire meals, for guests within days of a baby's arrival). But over the last twenty years Mongolia has undergone rapid urbanisation and economic growth and, consequently, there has been a change in infant-feeding habits, including an increase in the availability and use of formula. I was surprised by the most recent figures available, which show 50 per cent of infants in Mongolia are exclusively breastfed, placing the country below Sri Lanka (85 per cent), Cambodia (65 per cent) and India (55 per cent).[9] The arrival of the internet and easy access to homogenised online porn have shifted cultural attitudes towards breasts too. It is evidence of the ways social and economic changes impact methods of feeding children. While breastfeeding is still normalised in Mongolia, not everyone breastfeeds for great lengths of time any more; and yes, some can't breastfeed, but often this is due to socioeconomic reasons.

Thinking about differing cultural attitudes and maternal experiences can be productive and enlightening. Looking elsewhere can draw attention to the lack and deficits, a useful benefit in driving campaigns for change. It can help us imagine and advocate for better support for parents, imagine worlds where families are not atomised and breastfeeding is not taboo. But when these accounts become mythical narratives that exclude cultural and social nuance, they can instead function to make women feel guilty about their own experiences.

While the experience of learning to breastfeed often felt isolating – even with the wealth of support available to me – I knew, deep down, that my situation was far from unique. As I expressed milk or made up a bottle of formula, I would sometimes think of what kind of circumstances I might have found myself in had I been born in a different time or in another place. I wondered what options would have been available to me. I needed community, to thread myself into a network of parents and supporters, of joined-up government support. What I found instead was imposition and authority, which left me further fractured.

Part 3

THE ORDERED MOTHER

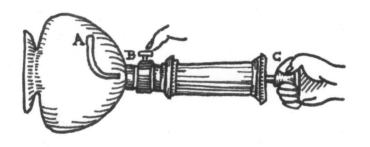

CHAPTER 7

Imposing Order

Smokey eyes, ringed with black kohl rather than sleep deprivation. Red lips, slightly parted, and hair artfully slicked back. A diamond Bulgari necklace framing the delicate collarbones, and a bright Versace jacket slung over the shoulders. From the black lace bra protrude two breast pumps, each between a quarter and a third full of milk. This is the photograph of actor Rachel McAdams that graced the cover of *Girls. Girls. Girls.* magazine in 2018. This photograph marked another moment of highly glossed celebration and visibility for parents who pump. Just months before, model Valeria Garcia had walked the runway while wearing a hands-free pump tucked into her bra. The realities of pumping or expressing milk were finally centre-stage. It felt, during my bleary-eyed night feed as I scrolled past the image of McAdams, like a moment of triumph.

The following day, slumped against the sofa, I began my own ritual of expressing milk with my manual pump. For all the photographs of women pumping while at a photoshoot or walking the catwalk, none captured the fraught physical and emotional labour that my pumping involved. There was no glamour here. Instead, I flailed around with the device, unsure how to use it optimally and constantly anxious about whether I was producing enough. The amounts seemed pitiful as I grimly measured against the graduated markers, drop by drop. As I pumped, I scrutinised the weight chart in my son's sacred red book. My finger followed the line from his birth down into a gully, then up to a peak at two weeks old, until the line sharply descended again. I obsessed over centiles.

Today, I open the 'red book' with the uncanny sense I get when visiting archives. I remember being told on our hospital discharge that we must keep it safe for twenty-five years. I remember a mix of panic and incredulity: I've just been given a helpless person to look after, and now you want me to look after this flimsy book too? Now, I pull out all the papers from the clear plastic wallet on the inside cover: one postcard illustrating how to hand-express; one laminated concertina about meningitis; the administrative birth notification; a blank piece of card; a letter from a lactation consultant for our GP; hospital discharge notes; a twelve-month development review questionnaire; four pages of colourful Comic Sans local health visitor information with phone numbers that had already gone out of service by the time my son was born. I can't breathe. I turn to the birth chart. There is a concentration of weight markers in the first three months and then the gaps between weigh-ins get longer, the jumps between centiles get higher.

Now I'm no longer in the trenches, I can see the logic in the feeding regime the hospital placed us on. Feed from the breast for a prescribed period; top up with an amount calculated by his weight (we scrawled the mathematical formula and calculations on scraps of paper); express a precise amount of milk from my body for the next 'top-up' bottle. I would feed my son, meticulously timed on a new app on my phone, pass him to his dad while I sat on the carpet, back propped up against the sofa, facing out towards our bay window. There was a steady rhythm to it, a predictability, and it ensured my son gained weight, little incremental increases in grams neatly plotted on the graph. I started to produce quantities of milk faster. I'd shout my results across the flat and my partner would peek round the door to give me a thumbs-up.

But if numbers gave security, they also left us doubting *me*. When everything is reduced to a number, what is unmeasurable can fall short. We all felt it. I sensed it when my partner asked if we could just give the baby a 'top-up' of formula, because he was, deep down, worried that our son was still hungry. The words were said with kindness, as much for me as for our son, but his question hit my ears as an accusation: he doesn't trust me. Doubts leaked into the rest of my being; what else was I unwittingly doing wrong? I felt like I was walking on a knife-edge; what could give reassurance and confidence was, at the same time, eroding the very same. My relationship to my body was unstable; it was an unreliable witness and creator.

I look back at the glossy Rachel McAdams photograph. All this celebration and visibility is wonderful. But, I realise, it has an unintended knock-on effect: another seed of doubt. In normalising the experiences of a lactating person, these images also distort our understanding of what normal *is*. I don't mean the aesthetic realities of pumping milk. Of course, we know that beyond the high-fashion hair and make-up, most people will pump on the sofa, in a toilet cubicle or hidden in an airless office. What I mean is the way cultural stuff causes us, collectively and individually, to distrust our bodies. There are long histories of women's bodies being doubted, our pains belittled, dismissed or ignored, particularly those belonging to women of colour. This is true of breastfeeding, where the acceptability and levels of societal interference in breastfeeding wax and wane, often in relationship to prevailing ideas over the institution of motherhood.

Few medical texts from the pre-modern period make more than passing reference to diseases relating to children, let alone mention their care in infancy. When reference is made to breastfeeding it is usually to note that women who nurse tended to have fewer pregnancies; a contraceptive effect that would have been as beneficial to men as to women. But by and large, infant care was a sphere from which men excluded themselves. In western Europe, the terms 'midwife', 'wet nurse', 'godmother' and even 'woman' could be interchangeable, as women's medical practices were a result of their daily lives *as women*.[1] Yet by the early modern period, the masculinisation of gynaecology had also seeped into infant care. In part this was due to a mistrust of midwives, who were privy to the mysteries surrounding birth and with knowledge of contraception and abortion. I began research into this period, stacking books and articles on my desk. One morning, I idly open one of the books and, as I flicked through the pages, I paused and blinked. Two disparate threads in the story of breastfeeding braid together unexpectedly for, it turns out, one of the most prominent figures in the European medical and cultural shifts around childbirth bears the same name as the twentieth-century artist who criss-crosses this book: Louise Bourgeois. This Bourgeois was a midwife and writer who straddled two distinct ages of midwifery. At the time of Bourgeois' birth just outside Paris in 1563, many women worked as midwives, offering neighbours assistance as needed. This may be how Bourgeois began her career. But she was also part of a wave of midwives to obtain official licences from the city of Paris, passing the official examination giving her a licence to practise in 1598. She worked alongside male physicians who were taking an ever-increasing interest in obstetrics, although Bourgeois earned a stellar reputation in her own right. Her official status as a midwife allowed her to attend aristocratic births and increase her income; she delivered all King Henri IV of France and his wife Marie de Medici's six children. Bourgeois was an advocate for scientific medical knowledge, the professionalisation of midwifery, and the importance of cooperation between surgeon and midwife. She published five works on midwifery, including *Recueil des secrets,* which contained recipes to cure various medical problems. But she also cautioned against unnecessary interventions from physicians during labour, and feared patriarchal control of maternity encroaching into physical birthing spaces.

The process of requiring midwives to obtain a licence was part of a Europe-wide movement to regulate the profession and bring them under greater state control. At the same time, male physicians were seeing an opportunity to expand their practice among the middle classes by moving into obstetrics. Although they were motivated by the aim of improving health outcomes for women and children, this also offered an increased market and potential for additional income. State intervention in birth and mothering resulted in a raft of changes in the eighteenth century. Lying-in hospitals were set up across Europe, providing sites for clinical education, training and experimentation, as well as somewhat safe havens for unmarried mothers. Women were to give birth in bed, which was more convenient for the male midwife. Outside of the birth room, men also began to publish works on how best to care for children. These manuals offer glimpses of the prevailing wisdom of the day, as well as charting the shift from women sharing knowledge – largely orally – to written instructions published largely by men. Less and less value was placed on maternal expertise, garnered from lived experience. Instead, manuals were part of an increasing trend for men to insert themselves into the previously feminine sphere of birth and infant care. Moreover, they resulted in a new sense of imposing order on the perinatal body.

State regulation of midwives was mirrored by attempts to regulate motherhood and this extended into the methods of feeding babies. Medical language approached the body as a machine and the reader as someone to be talked down to. As historical documents, for my purposes, these publications tell us less about infant-feeding practices than they do the prevailing discourses on maternity and femininity, the construction and reconstructions of ideas of 'the good mother'. The intended audience for these publications was most likely wealthy women, who were more likely to be literate but less likely to have access to inter-generational knowledge on breastfeeding, given that their mothers and grandmothers would have likely hired wet nurses. Less well-off women would have largely continued to rely on knowledge passed down from their mothers, other relatives and neighbours. Parallels can be made with the UK in the twentieth century, where trends towards infant formula meant there were generations of women who lacked first-hand knowledge to support their own daughters' breastfeeding journeys.

The first publications aimed at a female audience were keen to stress the health benefits of breastfeeding for mother and child. While there was the very real and urgent issue of high infant mortality rates, breastfeeding was also encouraged as part of a woman's natural and moral duty. Within this context, the term 'natural' meant wholly pure, good and harmless, rather than encompassing all that is bad and harmful that is also found within the natural world. One of the first and most influential books was published in 1748 by Dr William Cadogan, who at the time was working at the Bristol Infirmary. *An Essay Upon Nursing, and the Management of Children* was compiled not long after the birth of his daughter and took the form of a letter addressed to the Foundling Hospital in London, which had been founded by Thomas Coram a decade earlier. Cadogan begins with the words, 'It is with great Pleasure I see at last the Preservation of Children become the Care of Men of Sense'.[2] According to him, women lacked the learned knowledge of nature or philosophy required to adequately provide care for babies. Despite this, much of his advice itself was not unsound. In fact, Cadogan advocated breastfeeding babies for at least a year and waiting to give infants solid food until at least three months old. He also encouraged placing babies at the breast soon after birth to benefit from colostrum, rather than be fed any other foodstuffs at birth.

The book marked a turning point in infant-feeding practices. It was significant that Cadogan addressed his publication to the Foundling Hospital, who sent some babies out to wet nurses in the Home Counties while others were dry-fed with pap mixtures. A horrifyingly high number of babies died for want of adequate nourishment. This tragic fact was widely known among wealthier families in London, who, by the late eighteenth century, were visiting the hospital in large numbers, as a result of the public profile of patrons such as artist William Hogarth, who exhibited work there. In fact, thanks to support from artists the hospital became London's first public art gallery. When Cadogan was elected Physician of the Foundling Hospital in the 1750s, he moved between dinners with Sir Joshua Reynolds at David Garrick's house and the filthy streets of London where babies were still abandoned by terrified mothers.

Cadogan's essay struck a chord with William Buchan, a physician at the Foundling Hospital in Yorkshire, Buchan later authored his own incredibly influential medical handbook aimed at a general audience. Published in 1769,

Domestic Medicine was so popular it ran to 142 editions and was translated into many European languages. Buchan was also an advocate of breastfeeding, not only for the immediate benefit of babies, but also as a means to prevent health problems in later infancy. He was aware that there was, at that time, no adequate substitute for maternal milk, and saw that breast milk appeared to offer protection against childhood diseases, which babies fed by other means seemed less able to overcome.[3] Meanwhile, men started to publish memoirs in which they blamed their adult ill-health on their wet nurses, who came from the lower classes and who their former nurslings subsequently felt were less diligent and of lower moral standing. In the 1790s, medical doctor Hugh Smith published his *Letters to Married Women on Nursing and the Management of Children*. The book was intended for women, and he begins by explaining his use of the epistolary form as the most suitable for 'ladies' who would already be familiar with the style. He was concerned by infant mortality rates and included devastating tabulations in his publication. He urged women to breastfeed their own babies; yet reading his words now it is impossible for me not to roll my eyes when he writes 'the task is easy and delightful, and the thriving child rewards your pains. It is not laborious.'[4]

This kind of remark plays on the mix of paternal care and patronising tones found in these medical texts. The theme of women's vanity emerges strongly too; women themselves are blamed for not choosing to breastfeed their children. Cadogan, for example, was less interested in addressing the economic and class-based structures that impacted women's parenting choices, but instead blamed women's sexual vanity for their refusal to nurse their own babies. This was a vanity that the male medical establishment believed they could flatter. Smith argued that suckling improves not only the health of the infant, but also the mother's beauty: 'their husbands have, with pleasure, acknowledged their improved charms'.[5] This idea took root and in 1799, an American magazine wrote:

> A woman undergoes a kind of happy metamorphosis, which almost renders her difficult to be known. Her skin becomes fine, soft, and fair; her features are refined into an uncommon degrees of sweetness, under the influence of this new regimen. The too-ardent carnation of her cheeks, tempered by the milky revolution, assumes a milder teint.[6]

Sometimes, there seems little difference between the messages from two hundred years ago and today. Take the controversial 2018 'Be a Yummier Mummy' posters, which were displayed in a London hospital before being criticised across the internet for featuring bodycon dresses and sky-scraper heels, pandering to a woman's perceived vanity by telling us we could get our figures back faster and have more money to spend on shoes if only we'd just breastfeed, goddammit. A BBC News article from 1999 reporting on Tessa Jowell's 'breast is best' campaign also helpfully noted that breastfeeding mothers get their figures back faster.[7] I have spoken to many, many parents and not one has ever mentioned weight loss as factoring into their infant-feeding decisions. Despite this, there is a long history of women's perceived vanity being used to sway them into one mode of feeding their babies over another.

One of the greatest contributors to modern European ideas of breastfeeding is the French philosopher Jean-Jacques Rousseau. He laid out his vision for raising men uncorrupted by society through the narrative arc of the protagonist in the treatise-cum-novel, *Émile, ou De l'éducation*, published in 1762. In the book, the everyday practicalities of raising a child intertwine with Rosseau's moral philosophy and he is at his most declamatory when talking about breastfeeding. He railed against swaddling babies and sending them to live with wet nurses. As he saw it, women feeding their own babies would result in moral reform, as it was closer to an idealised 'natural state' of affairs and the first practical stage of instilling a moral 'goodness' into mankind. And if women would be 'good mothers', then men would become good fathers and husbands. The intimacy and bonds forged by breastfeeding would strengthen the ties not only of the nuclear family, but also those of wider society.

Never mind that Rousseau placed the five babies he fathered with his lover in a foundling hospital, of which he later wrote 'all were placed in the Foundling's Hospital, and with so little thought of the possibility of their identification that I did not even keep a record of their dates of birth'.[8]

Émile had a huge influence on French Revolutionary politics, and there were whole festivals where women nursed their babies en masse, a real-world spectacle that matched the breastfeeding imagery employed by the French Republic. But *Émile*'s most profound legacy was part of a much quieter revolution, one that took place in the fleshy bosom of the family. More and more women began to feed their own babies. Marie Antoinette herself was a great proponent of maternal nursing, breastfeeding her own child for a reported eighteen days before she was discouraged from continuing. She nevertheless persisted in encouraging other women to nurse their own babies. Elsewhere, state jurisdiction over maternal bodies became enshrined in law. The Prussian Legal Code of 1794 required all healthy women to breastfeed their children, although the Code also states that 'it is, however, the father's right to decide on the length of time she shall give her breast to the child'. As in France, women were seen as having a maternal duty to society.

Sometime between 1795 and 1800, Johann Friedrich August Tischbein painted a family portrait that embodied the biopolitical ideal of maternal breastfeeding. When I first saw the painting, I was startled by its composition and colour palette, noticing how the baby's red cheek had a flush that matched the mother's. The family scene takes place beneath a group of trees, green hills rolling gently away behind the father, who leans over a mound of grass. A great deal of attention has been given to the foliage, but the image's studied naturalism belies the influence of images of the Holy Family. The father wears a black tailcoat, with a flash of red protruding from the lapels. She, on the other hand, is enveloped in a cloud of white, which merges into the pale pink of the naked baby. Although the man is separated from his family by the grassy hillock and looks out at us, not at them, there is still a comfortable intimacy between the three. This was a nuclear family unit, celebrating maternal breastfeeding.

Tischbein's painting forms part of a broader cultural output that depicted the bliss found in family life and the trend towards maternal breastfeeding. Fashions also changed to accommodate the trend towards breastfeeding. The woman in Tischbein's painting wears a dress especially designed for nursing, opening at the front. A satirical print from 1796, now in the British Museum archives, shows a fashionable London woman seated in a chair, while through the window we can see a carriage waiting for her. A young maid holds a toddler towards the seated woman's bare breast. The baby clutches the breast as it latches. The woman, perched on her chair ready to leave, is dressed for the world. She wears a turban with two long plumes rising from it, drawing the eye up to a painting hung on the wall showing a woman breastfeeding, clearly titled *Maternal Love*. But the woman in the picture appears to hardly notice her baby. She is at best ambivalent, and certainly impatient with the task at hand. Her high-necked dress opens at two slits at each nipple and the print's title reveals the connection between aristocratic breastfeeding and fashion: *The fashionable mamma, – or – the convenience of modern dress.*

Whereas the daily practicalities of motherhood were once something aristocratic women would have avoided by employing wet nurses, now women across social strata were being encouraged to embrace the responsibilities of embodied maternity. In practice, many upper-class women still employed wet nurses, yet the importance of affection towards children in their infancy and maternal love were taking hold among the bourgeoisie. As art historian Carol Duncan argues, there was a trend towards emphasising the joyous aspects of motherhood, including the 'sensual rewards' and pleasures of nursing.[9] In mainland Europe breastfeeding was promoted on the basis of advancing the nation, and in England motherhood was being sold as the most emotionally satisfying role for a woman. Breastfeeding was established as the greatest bringer of joy and moral virtue.

Puritanical religious reformers in England and America were refashioning the maternal image of womanhood, using religious rather than medical or state techniques of persuasion. In 1835, Margaret Janet Moore stated in her book *A Grandmother's Advice to Young Mothers* that breastfeeding is 'a duty ... which is pointed out by the Creator of all beings'.[10] Breast milk was already a deeply embedded metaphor for spiritual awakening, but now an increased emphasis was placed on the selflessness, love and nurturing of virtuous motherhood, itself an identity that was being sentimentalised. This is exemplified in the writing of seventeenth-century English and colonial religious leaders, who used breast milk as a symbol for divine love. Eternal bliss was analogous to the happy baby at his mother's breast and weaning was symbolic of helplessness and spiritual loss. Puritan minister Thomas Shepard likened eternal life to being 'laid in the bosom of Christ, when sucking the breasts of the grace of Christ, when you can go no further, though thou wert in heaven, for there is no other happiness there'.[11] On the other hand, women who did not breastfeed their own babies were characterised as unnatural, sinful and vain. Breasts were maternal and utilitarian. Sending a child to a wet nurse was seen as a sign of an unnatural mother, and this criticism was often directed at wealthy and middle-class women, who were seen to prefer socialising and maintaining a fashionable physique to the solid work of nursing.

Typically, these largely male-authored publications managed to vilify both working-class and elite women. The elite were warned against hiring a working-class wet nurse, as their 'savage Tempers and vile Affections' could have a corrupting influence on the child.[12] Yet these wealthier women were also castigated for not adhering to the image of the idealised, wholesome working-class mother, ready to take on the 'natural' task of nursing. By the Victorian period, women themselves had begun authoring manuals in ever greater numbers, as well as offering advice and recommendations in women's magazines. The general message was still that women avoided breastfeeding for reasons of fashion or frivolity and that mothers who did not breastfeed must be somewhat unnatural and cold-blooded.

(Even today, 'natural' is also too often evoked as a synonym for easy, a fallacy that numerous breastfeeding counsellors debunked for me. One reminded me that 'breastfeeding is natural like walking, not like breathing'; anyone who has watched a toddler tumble and trip will know it doesn't always come easy. Natural is a social construct.)

How babies are fed continued to be an issue of national and moral importance into the early twentieth century. As if mothers didn't have it hard enough, they were, in the interwar years, tasked with raising mentally resilient and 'well-adjusted' children capable of running an Empire. After the Second World War, breastfeeding was encouraged in order to ensure 'the collective emotional health of the nation'.[13] Healthy citizens of good character were needed to ensure the survival of the British Empire, and it was believed that this started with the milk they consumed as babies. Recounting these histories here, I am struck by the paradox that still stalks us today. Infant-feeding was considered a societal, moral and biopolitical issue. Mothers were deemed able to make decisions based on sound reason, albeit steered by religious, political and medical authorities. Yet as I read these publications, I want to scream: if women were not breastfeeding because they worried it might ruin their figures, who was dictating what a 'ruined' figure looked like? Ultimately, men, I'd imagine. And if breastfeeding was of such national importance, why, decades later, was it made much harder for them by the demands of industrialisation?

All of this contributed to a wider movement of 'scientific motherhood', whereby raising babies was something to be done under the expert guidance of doctors. And, as might be expected from a 'scientific' method, regulating and quantifying feeds was central. The 'natural' aspect of breastfeeding, so prized by Rousseau, was diametrically opposed to 'scientific' methods, and needed to be tamed. One way to do this was to regulate feeds by creating strict routines, instructing mothers to feed their babies initially every two or three hours, with one feed in the night that was to be dropped after a few months whether the baby wanted to or not. Mothers were instructed to pay attention to the clock and not the cries of their babies. Although not endorsed by all, feeding on schedule became common advice. Experts were keen for habit and rhythm to be introduced in babies, by 'training' their tummies to process food at regular intervals rather than 'coddling' them with on-demand feeds. For many writers, this regulation was also educational, instilling the right kind of character in a child: stable, mentally sound and industrious. While the term used was 'scientific', I tend to think of it as 'militarised' motherhood.

Central to all of this was Frederic Truby King, a doctor from New Zealand. He founded the Mothercraft Training Society in London in 1917, and had little interest in the agency of a mother in deciding how she might prefer to feed her baby. According to him, breastfeeding was a baby's 'birthright'.[14] He also advocated for babies to be fed every four hours. Not only would this train the baby and avoid overloading their digestive system, it would also free women from the burden of constant feeds.

I try to square this advice with memories of my newborn, rooting and snuffling, looking for food, yes, but also comfort. I realise Truby King never felt the lightning shoot through his swollen breasts when his baby cried. I try to imagine pacing the floor with a wailing baby, bra damp with milk, watching minutes tick by. Of course, many mothers would have tolerated it all, believing that it was all for the best. Others would have ignored the prevailing advice. But I keep getting stuck on what babies are thought to be within this world ... automatons whose feeding should be a mechanised process, where feeding becomes mechanical rather than relational? Where clock time is privileged over responsive dialogue between baby and caregiver? Was there something to be feared in this relationship between mother and child? Something potentially powerful which needed to be stymied? I browsed the American Maternal and Child Health (MCH) Digital Library, looking at pamphlets for new parents from decades gone by. I find copies of booklets written for parents by the United States Children's Bureau, part of the US Department of Labor. The first pamphlet dates from 1914, and I scroll through thirty-one digitised pages that detail everything from bedding to dressing, shoes to playpens, until I find the section on feeding. There is a firm tone; nursing women are advised on what to eat to avoid indigestion or constipation, and how much exercise and sleep to have (the recommendation of at least eight hours sleep every night seems wildly optimistic). Babies are to be fed 'by the clock' and should be discouraged from suckling for more than twenty minutes at a time. The pamphlet goes on to advise on 'artificial feeding', suggesting cows' milk is the best substitute, provided it comes from a healthy herd and is purchased in sealed bottles. Advice from the American Medical Association at the time recommended quantities of sugar and lime water be added to the milk, the ratio of which should be based on the infant's age. Instructions are given on making a home-made ice box to keep the milk cool. The dizzying density of the pamphlet makes me anxious.

By 1929, the pamphlet had been updated, complete with line drawings of chubby babies and joyless, strict schedules for a baby's 'daily program and habit training' that extended beyond feeding. These instructions displaced mothers from the rhythms of their babies and of their own bodies. Through regime feeding and the advice of experts, a different sense of time and order was being imposed upon them. What the ordering of motherhood into regimes elides is the labour and time involved in breastfeeding. But what even is time in those early weeks of new parenthood?

CHAPTER 8

In and Out of Time

Bare skin is fusing with the lime pleather chair, which I've placed in front of the window. The air in here is oppressive and the as-yet-unnamed baby squirms in my arms. I watch blue sky turn orange then pink before it settles into the deep sapphire of late-summer night. Unsettled, I'm dwarfed by the chair, the sunset and these new responsibilities. I've not been outside since I braced myself against the rough brick wall at dawn four days ago, with my partner's steady count guiding me up to the summit of a contraction and back down again. Small plastic water cups litter the room, but my thirst is never quenched. The rising and the setting of the sun are the only temporal markers that make any sense to me now. The wall clock is redundant; when they tell me the doctor will visit at 11 a.m. they may as well be telling me they will arrive in the year 3032. All attention is on my breast, the gentle pull, the fluttering tongue. Time slows and stretches, and I am beholden to the rhythms of feeds and sleep, like the ebbs and flows of the moon and tides. But unlike the lunar cycles, this is an irregular beat. Time is elastic. His cries can last aeons, whole lifetimes are lost to nursing, and I am the ouroboros in the churn of it all.

Linear time creeps in. I see the life of my son stretching out into the horizon, a ball of wool unravelling as it rolls into the distance. As he suckles at my breast, I run my finger across his tiny palm, surprised again by the softness. All I can think is: where will these hands go? What will they carry? What things will they touch that haven't yet been invented? Whose hand will they hold when he no longer holds mine? Will those hands be kind? Time is suddenly measurable in a way it wasn't before. How old will I be when he is ten? Twenty-one? Forty-five? Oh . . .

His fingers grip mine and my own absence comes hurtling towards me.

Why did I keep going when breastfeeding was so hard? There would have been no shame in stopping. Yet I realise as I write this that I simply couldn't cope with the grief of not breastfeeding. Partly because of everything I had imagined it to be when I'd pictured my future motherhood. But I also needed to feel connected to my baby at a time when, as a new mother, I felt very disconnected from the world.

What I understand now is the urgent need I had for my body to sustain his life beyond pregnancy. There was a physical continuity that I didn't want to disrupt, which began with the umbilical cord and placenta and then ran through my breast. Despite the physical pain and emotional toil of learning to breastfeed, feeding him also offered me an unexpected kind of healing, a way of soothing painful memories that cycled through me. There were my childhood ideals of motherhood, but now I join the dots and can see that there were more recent events that contributed to this need for continuity and connection. There was already an overwhelm of grief that I couldn't bear to add to.

To be brief: eighteen months before my son was born, death tore a hole through my family, the pain of which was as intense as anything I'd ever felt before. It was the smell of snot and salt, burning eyes, the fiery palette of autumn leaves, trees quickly denuded, then the blankness of everything. By the time my son was born this raw grief was no longer visible; it had mutated into a quieter heartbreak that had burrowed itself deep and settled into my bones. My pregnancy and the birth had been lights in what had otherwise been a very bleak time and the baby's arrival was a balm that spelled possibility. But there was more. When someone dies by suicide those left behind agonise helplessly, wondering over and over: what signs did I miss? What could I have done differently? And then there is the refrain that reverberates through me even today, one that emphasises bodily presence: I should have been there. If my presence could have intervened – a phone call, a visit – then maybe things could have been different. At that moment, my love didn't reach far enough to hold him on the Earth any longer. I couldn't feel redundant and helpless again. My body needed to be salvation.

Feeding from my body was a way to continue the close connection between me and my baby; I couldn't articulate this then, but I had a profound need to continue to build his flesh and bone with the milk created close to my beating heart. I knew this wouldn't last forever and, as the feeds lessened in frequency, I began to understand how our relationship would always be a constant negotiation between leaving and returning. This push-and-pull is why I still lie with my son until he falls asleep each night. It is a moment in our day where industrial time pauses – even as I keep one eye on the clock – and we reconnect, getting lost in time together. I stay for as long as he wants me, watching his eyes flutter and come to close. His immediate and obvious need for me is lessening, but his knowledge of my presence is enough to let him leap into the unknowns of sleep. During the day, I learn to sit back and not to hover over his little self as he crawls with a measured amount of confidence and

trepidation across the highest wobbly bridge at the playground. I once read that 'birth is not so much a separation
of mother and baby, as a realignment of self and other', and
the sentence stopped me in my tracks.[1] It was the first time
I had found a phrasing that captured how breastfeeding felt
for me: a slow and gradual unfurling of our fates. I am very
aware that I can't save my child from time, but my body can
at least stave time off and be a place to regularly return to.
My body, the springboard for life. My milk.

I attempted to tether myself by logging time: work back
to calculate how little sleep we got, time our feeds, note
wet nappies, chart the baby's weight gain each day. Time
captured by measuring feeds and sleep, the stop-clock on
my phone, the alarm that wakes us in the night telling me
it's time to pump, the cycle of sterilising bottles after each
feed – also precisely timed.

Seven hundred and twenty hours and seven minutes.
This is how long one half of the Bristol graphic design duo
Conway and Young spent nursing her baby. You can check
the maths in *Milk Report* (2019), a slim, A4 zine with each
page divided into ten columns of biro-scribbled durations.
The baby's first feed lasted seventeen minutes. The last
documented feed – six months and four pale yellow pages
later – was precisely ten minutes. I can't help but admire her
commitment to keeping track and holding herself in time.

The report comes wrapped in a smaller, A5 publication,
printed on grey paper. It begins with Young's application
statement for the role of nursing mother; this is a job and
she outlines her experience accordingly. Young then takes
us to the hospital, where she notes her transformation into
a producer. In this role, the state monitors her efficiency,
refusing to release her and her baby home until they are satisfied that feeding is adequately established. Once released

into the world, she remains her own means of production, but the web of capitalism is still inescapable. If she is out and needs a place to feed, she will likely have to purchase something so she can nurse in a café. She must also purchase breast pads or nursing bras and, if she needs them, a nursing pillow, nipple cream, a breast pump, nipple shields, bottles and steriliser. None of which are available on the NHS. She notes statutory maternity pay isn't enough to survive on; 'so, as she unclips her bra again she is producing a person and replenishing the capitalist commodity of labour power'.[2] Her breastfeeding, even when feeding on demand, forms part of a larger economic and political order.

The *Milk Report* is priced at £8.21, the National Hourly Living Wage in 2019. A total of 720 copies were printed. If all sell, this will recompense Young £5,916.96 for her time spent breastfeeding. She can claim no expenses for any equipment purchased. There is no holiday or sick pay. There is no allowance for all the hidden labour her body does to produce milk between feeds.

If it seems too crude to reduce breastfeeding to monetary terms like this, then we are buying into a narrative that is centuries old and designed to keep women at a disadvantage. It is a narrative crafted from the idea that breastfeeding is emotionally satisfying and, moreover, our moral duty to our children and the nation. When wet-nursing fell out of favour, women were no longer paid for lactation and it became part of unpaid reproductive labour. Citing emotional fulfilment as the sole reward is a fantastic way of placing the burden of economic care onto the individual family unit. But emotions don't get us very far when we must pay the rent. Campaigns often like to remind women that breastfeeding is free, compared to bottle-feeding. But, as *Milk Report* starkly emphasised, breastfeeding is only completely free if you do not value women's labour and time.

And we can't help but log time. Count minutes, hours; work back to calculate how much or how little sleep we got; chart the baby's weight gain day by day. This is clock time. Sitting on that pleather chair in the hospital, I briefly thought back to an undergraduate course I took on metaphysics with the perfect stereotype of a British philosophy professor, who was so awkwardly captivating we gave him standing ovations. The only substance I really remember of those classes is the Scottish philosopher John McTaggart Ellis McTaggart, who argued that time does not exist. The specifics of his logic are lost to me now, but ever since that lecture I've thought about time differently, aware of how our division of time into segments of seconds, minutes, days, weeks and years is largely arbitrary. All time is contingent. And we often live within overlapping temporal registers.

If we were governed by the moon as much as the sun, we might have a better grasp of what Robbie Pfeufer Kahn has termed 'maialogical time'. This refers to the times of pregnancy, birth and lactation, which stand in contrast to the strictly linear sense of time that governs the West. Maialogical time is a temporality of interrelatedness, closely connected to bodily rhythms. It recognises that lactation can be akin to a mini-menstrual cycle, with hormonal fluctuations that ebb and flow from feed to feed. The bookends of our lives are often gendered as female, from the womb to burial in Mother Earth.[3] In her art, Louise Bourgeois circles back again and again to the maternal figure, with swollen bellies and breasts, sometimes titled *Self-Portrait*. She is cycling in maialogical time through into her nineties.

My breastfeeding world was governed by two temporal registers. One imposed order from the outside: clocks and growth charts, apps and timed feeds. It was all minutes and hours. The other was more responsive to my baby. I *knew* his weight was too low, even before I saw the numbers. Given I didn't have to balance the early days of breastfeeding with paid work, I was largely free to abandon myself to these cyclical rhythms. On days when I tried my best to ignore the feeding apps, passages of time were instead measured by how long I sat in the dark before my partner came home from work. An afternoon feed always turned into the baby napping on my chest, and I couldn't reach the lamp from the sofa without moving. Sleep, feed, change, repeat.

But then life in the twenty-first century creeps back in, with its own temporal demands. I spoke to several women who described the burden of managing multiple times: the clock-watching, diary-filled, email-checking alarm clock time of the post-industrial world contrasting sharply with the slow, regularly irregular and often cyclical rhythms of parenting. The return to paid work is having to live within these two temporal registers simultaneously, without letting one negatively impact the other. In an 'ideal' situation, one should not even know about the other; colleagues should never be made aware of parental temporality, of pumping in toilets, of hourly night feeds.

Regime feeding, while it certainly has its place, also imposes a particular sense of time on the lactating body. Ideas of frequency and duration, so dutifully recorded by parents in their own versions of *Milk Report,* ties time and quantity with adequacy and quality, as if parenting was akin to working in a factory. This comparison is more than a metaphor. In pre-industrial Europe, breastfed babies were usually fed on demand for at least a year, but societal changes that occurred as modernity swept the globe led to fundamental changes in how women fed their babies and how they understood their maternal bodies.

The introduction of industrialisation led to different conceptions of time and, in a world of factories and fore-men, timekeeping became crucial. At the same time, more women started to work outside of the home. This interest in the clock, in regimented time, combined with the interest in 'scientific motherhood', meant the medical establishment – predominantly men – encouraged women to stop feeding their babies on demand and instead feed them on a schedule. After the Industrial Revolution, the landscape of infant-feeding changed dramatically, particularly in urban areas, in line with the huge changes that had taken place across society. Breastfeeding rates in the UK varied from region to region, with the highest levels in rural and less industrialised areas where women could combine working from home with nursing their babies. But the rates were much lower in the industrial powerhouse areas.

Breastfeeding was affected by the kind of work a woman did, how far away it was from her home, and whether she had relatives nearby to help with childcare. For example, in the northern English mill towns of the Industrial Revolution, women would sometimes return to work just a few days after giving birth, leaving their newborns in the care of older sisters, aunties or older women within the local community. Sometimes a mother would breastfeed her child before and after work – doing the best that she possibly could – but during the long hours she was away in a factory the baby would be fed a range of alternative foods. While crèches were found across France, Italy and Austria from the 1840s onwards, which allowed mothers to breastfeed during their breaks, these were uncommon in the UK.

While physicians and philosophers called for more women to nurse their own babies for the sake of the health of society itself, the economic demands placed on families often made breastfeeding untenable. Industrial time was simply incompatible with and inhospitable to maialogical time. This shift to clock-watching, coupled with women leaving their babies for longer periods of time in order to work, negatively impacted milk production, which works on a supply and demand basis. Without the demands of a baby, individual women started producing less milk. This led women to doubt their own bodies and seek alternative sources of milk. Faintly repulsed by the plastic of baby bottles lined up fresh from the steriliser on a pristine tea towel on the kitchen table, I became fascinated by how women just a few generations before me would have managed.

Part 4

BOTTLES AND BREASTS

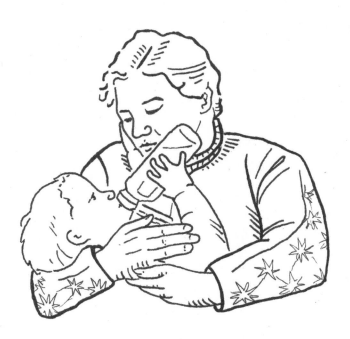

CHAPTER 9

Technologies of Feeding

Some 3,000 years ago, in an area now known as Bavaria, a bottle of milk was prepared for an infant. Made from pottery, it is a simple vessel, with an open cup and a narrow spout at the side. Another child is handed a more playful version, where the clay body has been given a stubby tail and animal head, complete with long ears and nose. The bodies of these bottles are small, perfectly sized for the hands of an infant. I picture hands sculpting the clay into the shape of a deer or a rabbit head, attaching it to the round bottle, and giving it little animal feet. I imagine an infant's giggles and gurgles, squidgy fingers reaching for the animal ears, pulling the spout to their lips as an adult hand guides the bottle so the fluid pours into the child's mouth and not over the ground. A fourth-century black-glazed baby-feeder from southern Italy has the words 'drink, don't drop' inscribed on the side in Greek.

How I wish I had known about these early bottles back when I was consumed with feelings of guilt for feeding my son from a plastic vessel. Of course bottles are not a modern phenomenon! Yet I had simply assumed baby bottles were a recent invention. Researchers have maintained this bias too, paying less attention to the technologies and 'social strategies' required in infant-feeding, labouring under the persistent yet erroneous idea that breastfeeding is simply a biological and physiological process.[1] Material culture was interpreted to have function besides the maternal and the familial. For example, when feeding bottles dating back to antiquity were first found in the Mediterranean area, it was thought they were used to hold other liquids, such as perfume or oil for lamps. Only when analysis of the terracotta pots was carried out in the 1990s was it revealed that they had once contained animal and/or human milk.[2] A recent study of bottle fragments found in Iron and Bronze Age infant burial sites in Bavaria confirmed that these vessels also contained traces of animal milk, belonging to goats, sheep or cattle.[3]

That these bottles were used to feed newborns remains a question. When bottles were used, it was more likely to wean slightly older infants. Given that lactation can have a contraceptive effect, weaning onto a bottle would help speed up a mother's return to fertility and allow her to reduce the gap between offspring. As the nomadic existence of the hunter-gatherer shifted to a life cultivating the land, the need for larger gaps between babies became less. It is easier to have a large brood of small children when you are settled in one place; much harder for a community to follow the seasons and the herds with many babies to carry. Isotopic evidence suggests hunter-gatherer children were breastfed until the age of five, while early farmers weaned their children at around the age of two or three. This move to an agricultural way of life also meant domesticated animals were on hand to supply supplementary milks. Such changes in weaning and feeding methods are also a reminder that infant-feeding is not only about individuals' situation, but that it also impacts – and is impacted by – how societies develop. And however unlikely it is that bottle-feeding babies was ever a widespread practice in prehistory, these fragments of pottery demonstrate how communities responded in emergency contexts, when things didn't go as planned.

Bottles continue to appear in the historical record. On display at the British Museum, in a gallery filled with vases, is a baby feeder from Sicily that has been dated to *c.*300 BCE. The ceramic body has been shaped into a mouse, with a spout for a tail. His legs are daintily tucked up beneath him and he has been intricately decorated, with delicate ears and carefully painted patterns. In the vitrine, the mouse sits beside an infant feeder shaped like a fish but with four unpainted fin-feet, which keep it standing upright. The body of the fish has been similarly painted black and decorated with white patterns and incised lines. A spout juts out above the tail.

The British Museum acquired the fish bottle in 1849, at the final sale of the collection of Richard Grenville, the 2nd Duke of Buckingham and Chandos and a politician, slave-owner and prolific collector. In 1847 he declared himself bankrupt. Such was the extent of his collection that the first sale of the contents of his palatial house at Stowe ran for forty long summer days. Other objects from his collection were acquired by the British Museum – Mughal miniatures, albums of calligraphy, satirical prints. I wonder where the fish bottle sat among it all?

And whose hands held this bottle? Did they wrap their fingers round the body of the mouse that someone crafted so beautifully? The hands that held these vessels, did they belong to babies who were being fed animal milk in a desperate attempt to keep them alive when no one in their community could? Had a woman manually expressed milk to fill the bottle because her baby couldn't latch on to her nipple? Even the earliest bottles reveal, with their incised decorative patterns and animal shapes, the love and the attention that went into parenting. But however much care went into crafting these vessels, they also had a darker side. They would have been difficult to clean, and bacteria would quickly flourish. Many bottle fragments have been unearthed at burial sites. At a site in present-day Sudan, two twin babies were placed side by side together with a small collection of tiny feeding vessels to sustain them in their next life. No matter how they functioned within communities, these bottles were also a parting gift, a last act of love to ensure the children remained satiated in their afterlife.

Whatever the circumstances, these babies were loved; someone was trying their best.

What bridges the gap between ceramic animal cups and BPA-free plastics? The collection in the Science Museum keeps me well occupied, albeit digitally via a screen because we are in the midst of a lockdown and all archives and museums have closed. But in my scrolling, I'm surprised to find, although I shouldn't be, pages and pages of infant-feeding bottles. Each click into another record reminds me that parents have always had to find technological and social solutions when raising their babies. Sure, many mothers can breastfeed without assistance, but there is a reassurance in knowing that I am not alone, nor is my body uniquely deficient. The more images I find, the more I ache for haptic connection. I want to reach through the screen and feel their weight, the cool of the glass and metal. I want to trace the touch of the last woman who used them. Was it her own baby she had been feeding? Or an orphan or a foundling? Each vessel, although now empty, contains a multitude of stories and emotions.

Given the uniformity of the modern-day, highly engineered baby bottle, the variety in forms of feeding vessels over the centuries astounds me. In one thirteenth-century French image, a woman recovers from birth while her attendants feed a swaddled baby, pouring fluid from a jug into an animal horn. In *The Poor Kitchen*, a sixteenth-century engraving based on drawings by Flemish artist Pieter Bruegel the Elder, scrawny adults fight over a bowl of mussels. In the corner, a gaunt woman feeds an equally scrappy child from a horn. The woman's breasts hang, exposed and limp, from above the bodice of her dress. In the engraving's counterpart, *The Rich Kitchen*, a corpulent woman sits in the centre of the epicurean scene with a chubby baby latched on to her full left breast.

One of the most striking objects I found in my search was a vertical bottle or jar made of ceramic by the Cahokia, the culture that used to extend across the Mississippi Valley and the present-day American Midwest. The bottle dates from between the thirteenth and fifteenth centuries. Recent scholarship suggests that women played a prominent role in Cahokian society; this is based on studies of statues of seated women interpreted as 'corn goddesses' or 'the old woman who never dies', a figure still central in modern Siouan-speaking tribes who are also located in the Mississippi valley.[4] The bottle that intrigues me is sculpted in the form of a seated woman nursing a baby. The spout appears at the top of the women's head. Was this a baby bottle? A ritual object? Whatever the bottle contained, whatever its function, the decorative feature of a breastfeeding woman shows the value the culture placed on this female task, perhaps linking the nourishing qualities of breast milk to the idea of abundance in corn crops.

In eighteenth-century Europe, curved glass and ceramic bottles borrowed the elegant horn shape. But now branding starts to appear, with 'Edward's' embossed in gold below an ornately carved wooden stopper. An eighteenth-century baby bottle from Germany was perhaps crafted with a child in mind. The glass is cloudy and painted with a colourful design of primary blues and yellows, with a sweet little invocation to 'Dinck nein karz liehef kind', which means 'drink, my sweet child'. I try to imagine a toddler holding this. I imagine the slightly sticky hands smearing the glass. But mostly, I worry about these bottles. I worry about them slipping and shattering; about babies throwing them from their cribs, shards scattering on the ground for other infants to pierce themselves on. I worry about cleaning them, about the dried yellowed milk caught in the delicate decoration of the glass. I worry about the temperature; the cold of the glass or the heat transferring too much too soon from warmed milk. I was a worrier before I became a mother and now the vigilance is sometimes too much to bear.

I am right to be concerned. Aesthetics were clearly a factor in bottle design, often unwittingly at the mercy of hygiene. These new materials were no better than pottery. Bottles made from pewter were dangerous as the milk absorbed the metals, which could poison the child. And the elegant organic forms in porcelain and crisp, cut-glass vertical bottles that wouldn't look out of place on a drinks cabinet were not easy to clean to a standard even close to sterile. Some Victorian bottles were so notoriously unhygienic that they gained the nickname 'murder bottles'. These were sometimes repurposed whisky bottles with long rubber hoses poked into the cork, which allowed infants to be left feeding unattended. The danger came less from the hose itself – ivory discs prevented the baby inhaling the nipple – and more from the impossibility of cleaning them. The inimitable Mrs Beeton only advised removing the nipple when it needed to be replaced, no more frequently than once a fortnight.

And as I examine these bottles, I become acutely aware of what they might have contained based on the period they date from. A dark, vertical bottle with a bulbous base and

curved spout dating from eighteenth-century England probably contained pap, that mix of flour or bread diluted in
water or animal milk. The bottle itself is made from pewter,
and every time I look at it I taste cold metal. Pap was commonly used alongside breast milk, as a means to wean an
infant or to liberate a mother from constantly nursing. Ale
or sugar was sometimes added to water down and sweeten
up these mucilages. Occasionally, the pap would be served
in a porcelain or metal boat, like a gravy dish, the designs
of which range from simple plain silver to decorative vessels
with vegetal repoussé, giving them visual and tactile interest.

The same eighteenth-century bottle could also contain
breast milk, drawn with a 'tire-lait', a breast reliever that
looks to me like a car boot sale knick-knack. I picture the
mother, early in the morning, her breasts heavy and full but
her baby, for whatever reason, unable to suckle from them
directly. She goes to the leather case that contains a glass
cup, like a small water tumbler with a thick, heavy base.
The cup has a concave cover, with a small hole at the centre,
into which she places her nipple. The glass is cold against
her skin and goosebumps cover her breast as the manual
vacuum pump starts to draw out the milk.

Had she lived a hundred years later, she might have
purchased her breast pump from S. Maw & Sons, who man-
ufactured pharmaceuticals and surgical equipment such as
post-mortem sets and vaginal syringes from their factory in
Aldersgate Street, London. She might have bought a simple
breast glass, placing the long tube at the top of the bottle
into her mouth to create a vacuum to draw out the milk.
But perhaps she had the means to purchase the more
expensive version that came in two parts, stored within
two plush velvet-lined compartments in a mahogany box.
The brass breast pump, appearing like a syringe, in tandem
with the clear glass bulb, was used as a siphon to draw off

the milk. S. Maw & Sons also made relievers from glass and rubber. Mothers tended to use these devices if they wanted to feed their babies in public using expressed milk, or if they had trouble directly breastfeeding. But these breast pumps were very much *scientific* instruments; they came with clear, one-page instructions recommending that a 'little sweet oil' should be applied to the leather or piston, but there is no mention of what to apply to the mother's breast if the flange made her nipples sore.

Then, in my archival searches, I found the nipple shields, ivory and glass forerunners of the flimsy silicone versions I used for a time, when my nipples were shredded from improperly used breast pumps. They were recommended to women to help them nurse through any pain. One nineteenth-century manual advised fastening a calf's teat to an ivory nipple shield, and women were advised that the teat should be preserved between feeds in gin and re-placed every ten to fourteen days. I associate shields with a squalling baby clutched in one arm and a slippery nipple hat escaping my other hand's fingers; with panic and ur-gency. But when I imagine a woman of relative means in the 1920s, removing her lead nipple shields that she used to prevent leaks and to stop the nipple from flattening under her clothes, I picture a mother with grace and poise. I also know, though, that as she opens the cardboard carton and removes the small, discreet, bulb-shaped breast pump, her nerves are likely fraying and she is daily having to wash milk stains from her clothes. She places the cold glass flange against her breast and the milk starts to flow into the bulb. Then she transfers the milk to a glass bottle. Someone made a special trip to the chemist to purchase 'The Alexandra', a glass bottle made by S. Maw, Son & Sons (more relatives joined the family business over the years). This bottle came with a set of cleaning brushes, packaged together neatly in a rectangular box, with an image of a grand building, foliage and a young man on the front. Every time the woman sees it, it momentarily soothes her, signifying a prosperous future for any (male) infant who feeds from the straw placed in the rubber stopper of the bottle.

The chill of glass bottles, with their hard, unyielding spouts made from metal or chamois leather, is far removed from a soft, warm silicone teat, designed to squish. Ever since Elijah Pratt patented the first rubber nipple in 1845, technology has been trying to mimic the mother's body ever more closely. Bubby pots, named after an old euphemism for breasts, were designed in the late eighteenth century and look like teapots with long, thin spouts. The spout has multiple holes, to mimic the human nipple. It is no coincidence that the development of infant-feeding technologies aligned with the Industrial Revolution in western Europe and North America, as the management of women's time between home and work changed. By the early twentieth century, firmly in the modern era, bottles had become more practical and uniform. And, in addition to bottles mimicking the breast, manufacturers also attempted to mimic the milk. Immersing myself in the deep history of bottles with their traces of animal milk has reminded me that there is no breastfeeding without there being, somewhere, an alternative to mother's milk.

CHAPTER 10

Alternative Milks

In the world of myth, stories abound of babies abandoned in the wilderness, pressing on them a wild otherness that later distinguishes them from the rest of the human population. Alone, these babies often find nourishment and care by being adopted into animal groups. Animal milk provides a counterpoint to the monstrous behaviours of the humans in these tales.

According to Greek myth, Zeus' mother hid him in a cave to protect him from his infanticidal father. Alone, Zeus was nursed by Amalthaea, a nymph, who fed him goat milk. Amalthaea is sometimes represented as a goat herself, nursing the young god from her teats. Heracles, whose own breastfeeding from Hera created the Milky Way, had a son, Telephus. Some stories say this boy was suckled by a doe. In the Pergamon Altar, a frieze shows Telephus being suckled by a lioness. Amulius ordered Romulus and Remus, his nephews and the legendary founders of Rome, to be drowned in the Tiber River. Amulius had good reason to fear his nephews reaching adulthood, given he had murdered all of their male relatives and imposed chastity on their mother, Rhea Silvia, who nevertheless was later assaulted and impregnated by Mars, the god of war. Amulius' servants, however, took pity on the twins and instead abandoned them on the riverbank, where they were eventually saved by a she-wolf. This event is captured in a famous bronze, now in the Capitoline Museum in Rome; two infants sit beneath the wolf's teats, their heads tilted up to catch her milk. There is some debate as to whether this particular wolf dates to the Roman period or is later, but it is known that the brothers were later additions to this scene, their fleshy roundness contrasting with the wolf's sinewy frame. She stands alert, eyes wide and ears pinned back. Her jaws open slightly to reveal her fangs. Her expression is a familiar mix of protective and fierce mothering, but her pose is also unusual in its ambiguity. She is panting, perhaps snarling, and her kindness is represented as instinctual, almost accidental. Rather than reclining to feed, she stands as if caught in a moment and poised to run. She is ambivalent at best about these strange boys feeding from her, as if she is not even aware they are not her own cubs.

Nourishment from animals marks these two infants apart from other mortal, everyday babies, emphasising their otherness. The fierce she-wolf's act of kindness in nourishing the foundlings is a powerful counterpoint to the savagery of murderous men and rapist gods.[1] But in reality, humans have turned to mammal milk for thousands of years at least. Evidence from prehistoric bottles suggests animal milk was a part of the human diet, at least for older babies and infants. At other times, animal milks were distrusted, often due to lingering fears that the baby may absorb the qualities of the animal. Italian writer Paolo da Certaldo issued a stark warning that an infant 'nourished on animal milk does not have wits like one fed on women's milk, but always looks stupid and vacant and not right in the head'.[2] Wet nurses were often the preferred option.

But when wet-nursing wasn't possible, there are instances of babies being suckled directly by animals. A text from the early fourteenth century recommends feeding a child suffering from pulmonary tuberculosis directly from a cow's udder. Several eighteenth-century engravings show babies in foundling hospitals being fed by goats. This was a relatively common practice from the sixteenth century onwards in France, as syphilis spread across Europe and the risk of infected babies passing the disease to wet nurses was widely discussed by physicians. Consequently, alternative feeding methods were needed, and goat milk was found to have a better success rate than feeding infants with gruel. Suckling directly from the animal also decreased risks of milk spoilage and of contamination from dirty bottles. When Dr Alphonse Leroy visited the foundling hospital in Aix in 1775, he couldn't have known that it was bacteria causing catastrophic outcomes in babies fed with animal milk in unclean bottles; bacteria was unknown at that time. But he did conclude that it was exposure to air that spoiled the milk, and his solution was to have the babies feed directly from the animals. Leroy described the scene thus: 'Each goat which comes to feed enters bleating and goes to hunt the infant which has been given to it, pushes back the covering with its horns and straddles the crib to give suck to the infant. Since that time they have raised very large numbers in that hospital.'[3]

In a striking painting from the nineteenth century by Niccolò Cannicci, a woman and child are seated in a stable. A chicken pecks at the straw on the ground. A goat disappears into the shadows, but a small infant is clearly illuminated as she suckles from the goat's udder. A woman cradles the baby and smiles, the baby's hands entwined with hers. Cannicci gives us tenderness rather than callousness, a reminder that the circumstances that might lead to a baby feeding from an animal teat are multiple, and always done with the best intentions.

*

Unpasteurised milk. Pap mixtures of flour, bread and water. Bottles riddled with bacteria. No wonder that in the early nineteenth century, one out of three babies who were not breastfed would perish before their first birthday. It took until I was writing this book for me to realise that the formula I fed my baby is so called because the 'scientific' thinking of the nineteenth century led to attempts find safer substitutes to the alternatives people had been using. It might not be as perfectly designed as breast milk, but formula has a sometimes life-saving history.

Given the suspicion around colostrum in many cultures, a newborn would be nursed by another lactating woman within the community. Such traditions enabled the mother to rest after labour and reap the benefits of having a community of caregivers that could support and feed the baby and mother after the exhaustions of labour. Writing in the eighteenth century and in support of his argument that women should nurse their own newborns, the physician William Cadogan provides an insight into what avoiding colostrum looked like in practice. He writes, 'the child as soon as it is born, is taken from the mother, and not suffered to suck till the milk comes of itself, but is either fed with stronge and improper things, or put to suck some other woman, whose milk flowing in a full stream, overpowers the new-born infant, that has not yet learned to swallow'.[4] Unsurprisingly, given that they were unable to adequately relieve their engorged breasts, it was fairly common for women at this time to suffer a 'milky fever' on the third or fourth day after childbirth. When a post-partum woman experienced fever or illness, there were also concerns about transmitting disease through milk. In 1789, Mary Wollstonecraft's husband, William Godwin, wrote an unsparingly frank account of the circumstances surrounding her death the previous year. The writer and feminist had died from complications after childbirth, possibly due to the incomplete removal of the placenta and subsequent septicaemia.[5] The practice of mothers nursing their own children had grown in popularity among the middle classes of the later eighteenth century, thanks in part to campaigning by the likes of Cadogan, and readers of Godwin's memoir would not have been surprised by the expectation that Wollstonecraft would nurse her baby herself. However, it appears that the doctor feared she might pass her infection to her newborn daughter, Mary, via the breast milk. Godwin recounts that, 'On Monday, Dr Fordyce forbad the child's having the breast, and we therefore procured puppies to draw off the milk'. The use of puppies would at least have prevented further engorgement and infection in the breasts.

This tantalising and discomforting detail of using animals as a feeding technology was historically less than unusual. In the first century CE, Soranus of Ephesus recommended that a newborn should be fed by a wet nurse for the first twenty days, as the mother's new milk was unwholesome. To maintain her supply, the mother could be suckled by other animals.[6] Dutch physician Paul Barbette wrote in the late seventeenth century that engorgement could be relieved either with an ointment of marshmallow or using a 'Woman or Whelp' [puppy] to suckle.

Yet the dangers of alternatives to breast milk were well known, as evidenced by the enduring global practice of wet-nursing. Henri-François Gaultier de Claubry, a French physician, wrote in 1783 that pap is 'the most dangerous of all foods for infants [. . .] it has caused to perish a great number, or has rendered them infirm and diseased all their lives'.[7] Animal milk or mixtures based on bread or grain also had dire consequences. Between 1775 and 1796, 10,272 infants were admitted to the Foundling Hospital in Dublin to be dry-nursed using pap. Of these, only forty-five survived. That is, 99.6 per cent of the babies died. Their notes simply read: 'Death from want of breast milk'.[8] Thankfully, by the middle of the nineteenth century, now that dangers of pap were causing moral outrage male scientists were increasingly turning their attention to alternatives to breast milk. Early weaning, where solid foods were introduced as early as two months, was also known to be unwise. As one commentator wrote about women pre-chewing meat for their small babies, 'it is very astonishing, that Mothers, who are so fond of their Children, as to be quite mad with Love of them, are not afraid to murder them with so improper a food'.[9] Suckling directly from animals was also not an ideal solution. On a practical level it was difficult to maintain healthy herds. At a deeper level, the practice was too taboo to be embraced across the population.

By the mid-nineteenth century the rubber teat had been invented, a device much easier to clean than the metal spouts of before and, perhaps reassuringly, more akin to the maternal nipple. This went hand in hand with research into increasing the shelf-life of ruminants' milk, first through condensing it and then, in 1864, through pasteurisation – named after Louis Pasteur, who discovered that the process killed bacteria and reduced the number of pathogens. Pasteurisation became standard across Europe and America, alongside other technologies such as refrigeration and sanitised packaging. In addition, advances in organic chemistry and increased medical interest in the composition of breast milk meant greater attention was given to replicating human milk, by comparing the chemical composition of human milk with that of cows, goats and sheep. The idea initially was to find a product for clinical use in emergency situations or to improve the outcomes for foundlings, rather than it becoming an everyday replacement for breast milk.

The scientific term 'formula' was used because it was a complex process and doctors would prescribe a particular recipe of ingredients based on a baby's needs. But the product would quickly become a commercial venture, unable to escape the grim, inevitable grip of capitalism.

The first commercial formula milk was launched in 1865. Liebig's Soluble Food for Babies contained cows' milk, malt flour, wheat flour and potassium bicarbonate and was advertised as 'the most perfect substitute for mother's milk'.[10] It had been invented by the German chemist Justus von Liebig, the son of a pigment manufacturer who spent his childhood in his father's small laboratory. He was thirteen when Mount Tambora, in Indonesia, erupted, which sent volcanic ash clouds westward, blocking the sun. The resulting blackout of 1816 was known as the 'year without summer' and von Liebig would have seen crops fail and food prices rise, as people were forced to eat grass and rats. As an adult, his work in organic chemistry, manufacturing nutritional foodstuffs for the infirm, as well as infant formula, was undoubtedly impacted by witnessing such scarcity. There is reassurance to be found in this honourable origin of a substance I once read described as 'poison'. At around the same time, chemist, inventor and merchant Henri Nestlé developed his own formula, which could be mixed with water. At least for those with access to clean water, resources to pay for formula products, and hygienic facilities to sterilise equipment, safer alternatives to breast milk were finally here.

By 1883, there were twenty-seven patented brands of infant formula. Soon companies began more aggressive marketing campaigns, positioning formula as more than a medical substitute. By the early twentieth century, formula companies were funding research to support their health claims. These tried to show that babies fed on evaporated milk formulas did much better than breastfed babies, based upon weight gain and those growth charts that haunted my early weeks of motherhood. Formula also benefited from savvy marketing. Being quantifiable, formula aligned with the move towards 'scientific motherhood'; amounts could be easily and reassuringly measured. Adverts showed plump, rosy-cheeked, blond babies, with their doting mothers and, in some cases, smiling doctors, reinforcing the endorsement by medical authorities. A 1930s advert, for example, borrows Renaissance madonna tropes, depicting a glowing mother dressed in blue feeding her chubby infant from a bottle, while another child at her knee looks up at her adoringly. Formula companies were keen to exploit families' worries and hopes for their babies, capitalising on the trend towards scientific and medical expertise that had displaced and undermined traditional female knowledge in the field of infant-feeding. Formula was branded as an upgrade on human milk and used evocative terms such as 'Gold' or 'Advanced'. One brand was even called Humanised Trufood. The messaging was clear: this product will improve the physical and mental health of your baby. One American print advert claimed babies reared on their product 'have the brain, brawn and sinew to develop the helpful men and women of the future'.

But this marketing proved massively controversial, and with good reason. The most egregious practices occurred in the 1960s, when birth rates in the West were in decline and companies began searching for new markets. In glossy adverts designed for consumers in the Global South, manufacturers homed in on precisely what any marketer knows: new parents are ripe for exploitation. Wanting the absolute best for their newly minted child, parents are a captive audience for aspirational advertising. Many communities in the Global South had deeply ingrained confidence in a mother's ability to produce sufficient milk for her child, but corporations were adept at planting seeds of doubt nonetheless. They used slogans describing formula as a 'modern' and 'scientific' product, positioning it as an aspirational item that any 'good mother' should want to provide for their babies. By dressing their sales reps as nurses, they used the cachet of scientific and medical expertise to entice mothers who had limited access to decent healthcare. These reps stalked maternity wards and urban areas, looking for the tell-tale sign of nappies hung out on the washing line.

In one of the most infamous examples, Nestlé benignly offered new mothers in the Global South free samples of their product. But, as we've seen, breast milk works on a supply and demand basis; once the mother had used her free samples, her own supply would have likely been reduced. Unable to continue breastfeeding, she would be forced to purchase the formula. If cost became an issue, as it so often did, parents would water down the powder to eke it out, lowering its nutritional value. And, because many families lacked access to clean water, formula was often mixed with unsanitary water, which had catastrophic consequences.

It is the highly questionable ethics of the companies that taints formula. As a politically precocious child of the 1980s, I grew up very aware of the Nestlé boycott that had begun the decade before. In 1973, the *New Internationalist* ran an article called 'Babies Mean Business', which accused Nestlé of creating need where none had existed. While Nestlé attempted to address these concerns, the newly formed International Baby Food Action Network campaigned for greater regulation of the baby formula industry. The WHO/UNICEF International Code of Marketing of Breastmilk Substitutes was established in 1981, designed to protect breastfeeding and restrict spurious marketing claims, ensuring that buyers were able to make choices based on unbiased, factually correct claims. Nestlé signed up in 1984. However, many companies in many countries still fail to meet the standards of this voluntary code.[11] The breast-milk substitutes market is worth, globally, $70bn per annum and companies find ways to exploit loopholes in the Code, spending $6bn a year on marketing.[12] For example, companies can promote toddler milks, allowing them to bypass the Code's restrictions on marketing formula for babies. Savvy branding means that families can end up feeling pressure to buy more expensive milks or 'follow-on' milk for toddlers, at a time when for most children cows' milk will suffice.

This points to a fundamental issue with public health campaigns: they must compete with expensive and aggressive marketing from formula companies. This marketing – under-regulated in some countries – can encourage women to doubt their own bodies by offering them a solution to problems that often do not exist. These tactics then force public health bodies to pitch themselves against the corporate advertising dollar, resulting in pithy campaigns that – out of necessity – lack nuance. Among all this, as long as infant formula is a profit-driven commodity, individuals the world over are the unwitting victims. As I opened a pre-mixed plastic bottle of formula in that hospital room, I felt as if we were now complicit in their immoral marketing activities. As if by ingesting their concoctions my son would be imbibing the moral qualities of the manufacturer. I had conflated formula milk with the formula milk industry.

There are new developments on the horizon in the field of infant-feeding, which bring with them new ethical questions. In June 2020, Bill Gates bought a $3.5m stake in Biomilq, the company founded by Dr Leila Strickland, a cell biologist and mother who herself eventually switched from breast milk to formula after experiencing myriad feeding problems. Dr Strickland discovered how to develop breast cells in the lab and collect the milk they produce. In June 2021, Biomilq announced they had successfully produced the 'world's first cell-cultured human milk outside of the breast'. Yet the company itself acknowledges there are components and qualities that the lab-produced milk cannot replicate. The milk won't adapt in response to the baby's needs in real time, nor will it contain hormones, bacteria or antibodies, which all enter the milk via the mother's bloodstream. But beyond its composition, there are other fundamental issues at stake. On the one hand, this biotechnology offers parents potential freedom of choice and better alternatives. This is to be celebrated. Yet nothing is neutral in this sphere. Torn on the potential benefits of lab-grown milk, I also fear that these kinds of developments could lead to the rollback of many of the hard-won concessions currently available to new parents. In the UK, for example, extended maternity leave is legally mandated and employers are required to provide space and facilities for mothers who need to express milk during the working day. If breast milk could be purchased in the supermarket, what would happen to the need for support and flexibility for lactating parents?

When I asked mothers their thoughts on lab-produced breast milk their responses mirrored my own: grateful that research into breastfeeding was being carried out, cautiously optimistic for an alternative to formula, all mixed with a weary dose of scepticism. Several expressed concern that the product could become another stick to beat new parents with. What happens if, like me, you have to 'top up'. Do you feel ashamed if you can 'only' afford powdered formula, rather than lab milk? Everyone I spoke with feared the latter would be given a heavy price tag, creating yet more division and more guilt. As one British mother said, 'In an ideal world this would be just another tool for parents to feed their babies, but we all know it's much more complex than that; it stirs debate about women's bodies and what they choose to do with them.' When it comes to reproductive technologies we need to 'both honour women's bodies and enlarge the availability of (women-centred) options for those who cannot have or do not want the embodied experiences'.[13] Lab milk as well as the sophisticated and discreet breast pumps now on the market are only an advance for feminist parenthood when they are truly accessible to all. Equality of access to these technological developments is key.

Like everything in late-stage capitalism, nothing is free from globalised exploitation. Technological developments in infant-feeding have been driven as much by profit as public health concerns and are therefore vulnerable to the ethical issues faced by other global industries, such as fair working conditions and pay. In 2017, the Cambodian government banned the sale and export of human breast milk after an increasing number of reports suggested that women were being exploited by for-profit American companies.[14] Utah-based Ambrosia Labs was one such company; it sourced breast milk in Cambodia to distribute across the USA, where it sold for $20 for 147ml. The women in Cambodia were reportedly paid between $7 and $10 per day, which is around twice the rate of pay for a female construction worker (Cambodia's official minimum wage is $190 per month). UNICEF described the practice as 'exploiting vulnerable and poor women for profit and commercial purposes'.[15] Yet, some of the women paid for their milk noted that the work allowed them more time with their own children and better pay compared with alternative sources of income, such as long shifts in garment factories. How do we untangle exploitation from autonomy? Paternalism from protection?

Elsewhere, other economies are at work. Globally there are just under 800 milk banks, fifteen of which are in the UK. These screen and pasteurise donated human milk before passing it on, often to nourish low birth-weight and sick newborn babies. And, beyond milk banks, women also informally donate breast milk to friends or feed one another's babies. I know of one group of women who each expressed breast milk to give to a friend. She was struggling to establish feeding in her new baby but didn't want her child to miss out on the important benefits of breast milk. When one of these informal donors confessed this to a health visitor they were reprimanded. Ostensibly this was over fears of passing on HIV or AIDS, but maybe the health visitor was squeamish about the idea of shared feeding or a baby drinking another woman's breast milk. These informal groups of parents exchanging breast milk excites me; it seems like a quiet form of anti-capitalist activism, building communities of mutual support.

Alongside milk and nourishment and bonds, there is always politics.

Part 5

THE POLITICS OF MILK

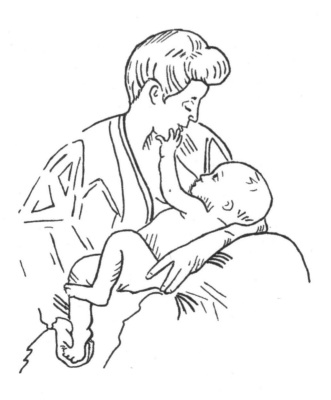

CHAPTER 11

Being Seen

A Spanish mother of one told me that, for her, 'breastfeeding is about comfort, some sort of home. It is also part of the mother's sexuality.' I marvelled at the simplicity of these words. I also marvelled at their weight. Breastfeeding is about more than just the milk, more than just a baby and a breast. History shows us how trends ebb and flow, how attitudes to mothering bodies shift, how we are all caught in webs made of many threads. Breastfeeding is never apolitical, 'given the way it positions women's bodies in relation to infants and partners, the issues it raises for women in public spaces, and how it forces a reconceptualisation of the idea of the autonomous individual that is the basis for Western conceptions of the civic polity and, thus, citizenship.'[1] And we can't talk about milk without talking about bodies that produce and consume: their presence, their absence, their replication.

I have a postcard pinned beside my computer that I bought from Dulwich Picture Gallery when my son was a few months old. By this time, any nerves I had about getting him to latch successfully in public had vanished. My flow had regulated itself and I had mastered the art of discreetly arranging my clothes. The postcard is of a painting by Peter Paul Rubens from around 1635, and it continues to hold my attention for its celebration of milky bodies. The figure of Venus cuts through the centre of the image, a luminous rippling body, naked but for a Marian blue cloth held across her upper thighs, and a wisp of translucent fabric caught across her right shoulder. Her right hand sandwiches her left breast, scissoring the nipple between her fingers so that jets of white milk arc towards the open mouth of Cupid, who sits beneath her balanced on Mars' sword. The child clutches Venus' arm to prevent his naked body from falling. Mars, the god of war, dark against a backdrop of bloody red brushstrokes, looks down towards the boy with a brooding softness.

Moments before buying a postcard of this allegorical image of love winning over war, with such attention given to the fleshy reality of hand-expressing milk, milk that streaked across the canvas, I had seen a wrinkle of discomfort skim across the face of a woman in the gallery café as I opened my nursing bra. I was alert to my surroundings in the way that new parents often are, especially those about to breast-feed, as they negotiate new and familiar spaces, unsure what the 'rules' are or where the borders between public and privacy now lie.[2] These new codes are made more confusing because of the way breastfeeding bodies are celebrated and also censured, revered yet viewed with discomfort.

Ideas of what constitutes public and private spaces shift and evolve over place and time. In the West, industrialisation and urbanisation saw work firmly separated from the home, and the latter became viewed as a largely female domain. By the end of the nineteenth century, British mothers were being castigated for leaving their babies in order to go out to work in factories. In effect, they were blamed for the social and economic structures that disempowered them, pushed them into paid work, and then admonished them for doing so. But this social and gendered division of labour meant that breastfeeding bodies were no longer as visible as they would have been when work and domestic life were folded in together.

This new invisibility extended into the home as well. In the fifteenth and sixteenth centuries in England, houses were designed as an interlocking series of rooms so that one would need to move through one bedchamber to get to another. This was true even in the great homes of the wealthy. But attitudes towards privacy changed, and by the end of the seventeenth century bedrooms were moved upstairs and rooms were linked by hallways. This increased sense of privacy trickled down to smaller, more modest homes, whereby spaces were divided up according to function.

Beyond the house, the idea that one needed to behave in a 'civilised' manner filtered through Europe. This concept of civility started to impact how people thought about their dress, their personal hygiene and their body and its functions. More and more, real-life lactating bodies in Europe were hidden from view.

Breast milk joins two bodies, one incorporated into the other; the boundaries of the individual body are blurred, which offers a partial explanation for our present cultural discomfort around breastfeeding, especially beyond the newborn stage or in public. I suspect this coupling of bodies makes people uneasy, particularly in a Western patriarchal society where identity is founded on the sovereign individual and where our societal attitudes towards sex are similarly confused and contradictory. Indeed, in the early twentieth century, breastfeeding formed one of the earliest phases in Sigmund Freud's psychoanalytical theory of psychosexual development. In this theory, breastfeeding too much or too little, weaning too early or too late, all had the potential to result in sexually maladaptive adult behaviours.

As I explore later in this book, we are culturally confused

and limited in our attitudes towards nursing and sex, the maternal breast and the sexual breast. However, psychoanalysis offers another angle for thinking through other latent cultural taboos which blight breastfeeding. In the 1980s, Louise Bourgeois staged several performance works where her models wore robes adorned with latex globules. In *A Banquet/ A Fashion Show of Body Parts*, a long table stretched the length of the catwalk, replete with bulbous, fleshy lumps. Bourgeois was well-versed in the work of Melanie Klein and this artwork can be read as a response to psychoanalytical ideas of the breastfeeding body. Klein was an early follower of Freud and focused on infancy, examining the centrality of the body of the mother – specifically her breasts – in childhood development. Klein's work was novel in that she recognised the emotional, as well as physical, needs of the newborn baby. Her 1936 essay 'Weaning' widened Freud's concern with breastfeeding and sexuality into a broader interest in how infant-feeding could impact the future well-being of the child. The previous worries over the kinds of humoral and temperamental qualities a wet nurse may pass on to a child through her physical milk shifted towards what kinds of emotions and ideas are formed at experiential and unconscious levels. The maternal breast is an object central to the infant's fantastical imaginings and their heliocentric narcissism, with the child, according to Klein, imagining they are consuming and possessing the flesh. Bourgeois' banquet plays with ideas of women and food, breasts and consumption, confronting the cannibalistic imagery that lurks in the shadows of our cultural milieu. Babies eating from our bodies, our parasitical progeny. Maybe this is why public breastfeeding is such a vexed topic?

I fed my baby everywhere, primarily because if I was in public and my baby was hungry then I was determined to feed him without shame. But I knew doing so could cause controversy, aware as I was that I had internalised a sense of shame that I now had to rebuke. A quick search of news articles from the last ten years shows reports of numerous cases of women being asked to move elsewhere or cover up while publicly breastfeeding, followed by breastfeeding sit-in protests in response. This has happened on the Gold Coast in Australia, at a swimming pool in Minnesota, at the Museum of Modern Art in Mexico City (the woman was asked to leave as the museum forbade drinking in the galleries).[3] This drip-drip of media articles continually re-inforces the precarious position of nursing in public. And it is not only the physical act of nursing that is open to cen-sure. In 2011, a gallery in Warsaw pre-emptively cancelled an exhibition of entries to a photography competition or-ganised by a pro-breastfeeding organisation. In explaining the reasons for cancelling, the gallery cited fears of potential offence to gallery audiences, although the precise cause of the offence, and to whom, was not made clear.[4] Follow-ing the news of this decision, roughly 200 women staged a public breastfeeding protest at a Warsaw metro station. Some attendees nursed their babies, others held up religious paintings of the *Madonna lactans*, highlighting the hypoc-risy of censoring contemporary breastfeeding imagery on potentially religious grounds. The protest was covered by local and national news outlets, which predictably sparked fierce debate in online comment sections. Some commenta-tors were supportive, others disputed the artistic merit of the photographs, while others still expressed abject disgust, likening breastfeeding to public urination or defecation. Some referred to the women who attended and breastfed their babies publicly as exhibitionists.

Most cisgender women I spoke to felt generally com-fortable nursing in certain public spaces. Very few reported overt hostility, such as when a friend of a friend was called a 'dirty slag' for breastfeeding on a bench in Brighton (of all places). But all shared stories that describe a slow grind of small doses of disapproval. The staring, double-takes and tutting. Disapproving looks and muttering. All minimised the experience, saying they felt 'lucky' not to have met more outright discrimination. There is stoicism: my baby must be fed, so screw you.

Yet we all know that, from coffee-chain employees demanding patrons breastfeed in the toilet to Facebook evoking its own obscenity rules when its algorithm removed images of breastfeeding mothers, the nursing body is subject to scrutiny, censorship and discrimination.[5] Breastfeeding can be a provocation, an armour built of vulnerability as well as life-giving power, and, for me, breastfeeding in public felt like a political act. However broken I felt in my new motherhood when in public I always felt an enormous power in my lactating body, liberated as it was from the sexualised male gaze. I was glad if some people found breast-feeding distasteful; if they harboured a discomfort at seeing a woman use her body for something other than to please the rest of the world, then I wanted to provoke it. Some-times I willed a person to make a negative comment just so that I could blow off steam and release the simmering anger that was collecting in my sleep-deprived, hormonal, anxious brain. I breastfed in pubs and on the kerb outside pubs and in a window seat in Caffè Nero on Tottenham Court Road, while passers-by stared at me like a performance art exhibit. This was a necessity, but it was also quiet activism.

I breastfed at a Mothers Rise Up march against climate change, feeling transformed by my maternal status, which lent me a greater urgency in addressing catastrophic climate change. One lunchtime shortly after my baby's first birth-day, at a new job in Millbank, my boss gestured out of the plate-glass window to the ground below and told me how, two months before, a group of women from Extinction Rebellion had held a nurse-in. They had blockaded the road with their babies and breasts and potential taboos. I've seen the photos: a sea of mostly white women sat cross-legged in the road with babies of all ages laid across their laps and tucked under their shirts. A placard depicts a breast in profile, like a globe; a drop of milk falls like a tear from the nipple. *Please don't suck me dry,* it pleads. After the murder of George Floyd – who called for his life and his mother – a doula named Kyla Carlos attended a Black Lives Matter protest in Virginia, breastfeeding her newborn baby while holding up a power fist.

At the intersection of activism spectacle and community-building is American artist Jill Miller, who created a bold, visible marker of breastfeeding in response to a lack of safe public spaces for parents to nurse. In 2011, she raised $15,500 on Kickstarter for the purchase of an old ice cream van, which she converted into a breastfeeding support centre. *The Milk Truck* is unmissable, its cab decorated in large pink and blue polka dots, the back section in stripes of equally bold colours. The breast sits on its roof like a large pink blancmange, with a flashing nipple on top. Even the van's hubcaps are bright pink. The van is camp, kitsch and disarming and, driving through the streets of Pittsburgh, this multi-year project made the fact of breastfeeding inescapable to any passer-by. In her Kickstarter video, Miller envisages a van that responds to breastfeeding 'emergencies', to be called on when, for example, a woman nursing in a restaurant is asked to 'stop creating a spectacle'. The van arrives, providing a sanctuary for breastfeeding, and brings with it hordes of breastfeeding allies to stage a breastfeed-in within the offending premises.

The Milk Truck allows for a space for peaceful breast-feeding, while also making the whole thing spectacularly visible. This idea of revealing and concealing made me wonder how my body was viewed from the outside. I knew I had legal protections: the right to breastfeed is enshrined in UK law, under the Equality Act 2010. This protects the right to breastfeed in any public space, including on public transport, as well as in commercial spaces such as restaurants, cafés, shops and cinemas. Yet at least a third of the UK population think breastfeeding in public is wrong, and more people think it's preferable for a baby to be fed in a toilet than at a table in a restaurant, according to research by Professor Amy Brown.[6]

I've not run a statistical analysis, but I'd guess a significant percentage of media attention on breastfeeding is devoted to the countless breastfeeding sit-ins that have been staged across the globe, usually in response to someone being asked to leave a public space or cover up. These reports reinforce the idea that there is something 'controversial' about breastfeeding in public, presenting the issue as something open for 'debate' rather than something that should be protected by right. A case in point is the 2014 story of a Staffordshire woman secretly photographed by a member of the public while she stopped on the way home from the shops to breastfeed her baby on the steps of a closed pub. The photo was posted on Facebook without the woman's consent, under the caption 'tramp'. After she was alerted to the image online, the mother mobilised a campaign that saw groups of women congregate to breastfeed in public spaces across the UK.

This example raises several interlinked issues. The first is the protections afforded to public breastfeeding while also protecting the privacy of the nursing person (more on that in a moment). The second is that in the manner of reporting these stories, the mainstream media can make parents feel uneasy about public breastfeeding before they've even given birth. These kinds of viral stories can lead to a double shaming: the event itself that the article refers to and then the negativity such stories attract. Each media article is a reminder that the public sphere is not always accommodating to lactating people. Underpinning all of this are the culturally embedded power structures that give women – especially marginalised women and non-binary people – less agency and control in how they are represented. The result is that we accept graphic depictions of lactation in seventeenth-century allegorical paintings but feel unsure when it comes to breastfeeding in twenty-first-century cafés. The idea of a white cis woman breastfeeding in public is still framed as a polarising debate, so much so that the acceptability of the act was still open for discussion on BBC *Woman's Hour* in 2021. Any conversation framed as a debate surrounding breastfeeding in public suggests tacit acceptance of the idea of breast milk or the lactating body as taboo, unpleasant, unsightly or squeamish. A debate suggests that the call for parents to only to breastfeed *in private* is a tenable position.

Breastfeeding is censored elsewhere too. In 2014, Ashlee Wells Jackson's social media accounts, where she shared images from her 4th Trimester Bodies project, were deleted from Instagram nine times, usually without warning or explanation.[7] Instagram is notorious for having a ban on female nipples in photography, although those depicted in painting and sculpture are exempt. In response to this unofficial ban on breastfeeding, Jackson started the 'Stop Censoring Motherhood' campaign, doctoring her own images on social media with a black heart and slogan. In response to pressure, Instagram later announced it would allow breastfeeding images, but the ban on female nipples remains in place[8]. Even the Woman of Willendorf was a victim of Facebook's censorious algorithm, which in 2018 deleted a post containing an image of the statue as it was deemed 'pornographic'.[9] A spokesperson for Facebook later apologised for the error.[10]

Juxtapose this corporate ban on breasts with the fact that, in the UK at the time of writing, it is not illegal to take a photograph of a person breastfeeding without that person's consent. This was so shocking to me that I had to verify this multiple times. But it is true: the Voyeurism Act, passed in 2019, bans the taking of non-consensual photographs of genitals or buttocks – known as upskirting – but it does not criminalise photographs of the upper body. In May 2021, MP Stella Creasy launched a campaign to criminalise such acts of voyeurism after one of her constituents saw a man taking photographs of her while she was breastfeeding with other mums in the park. The man was using a long-lens camera and when confronted refused to delete the photographs. When the woman went to Greater Manchester Police, she was told no crime had been committed. Ms Creasy had also experienced being photographed on public transport by a teenage boy while breastfeeding her small baby.

If laws have been made to protect the right to breastfeed in public, the policing of our lactating bodies takes place beyond the state and instead lies in our media, our communities and our cultures. This policing extends to ourselves too. Several women I spoke to used the very term 'police' to describe their decision to stop breastfeeding in public when their babies reached a certain age. They felt that being seen nursing an older infant would be viewed as less acceptable, worrying that they might be more likely to experience overt public disapproval. But we also police our own reactions and responses; a woman who breastfed her child for almost two years described her performance of eye-rolls and grumbles of annoyance whenever she had to excuse herself from friends and family to feed her child. She feared their pity or judgement and therefore pre-empted it and tried to shut it down with her own exaggerated displeasure at the process. What she couldn't tell them was just how much she looked forward to those private moments nursing her child. She said breastfeeding was rarely an imposition at all. Yet her pretence was needed to make it acceptable to others.

I remember breastfeeding my son at a new-mother group, while the woman next to me produced a bottle from her nappy bag. Panic set in as I worried that she was feeling like I would judge her, or that I would be judged for making judgements.

Parents living with a constant sense of scrutiny, and media reports of parents who have been shamed, are a product of a broader culture of surveillance, where women are made to feel as if they are constantly being watched, compared and – usually – found lacking. Used to being watched, we in turn watch ourselves and each other, assuming we are all being judged; lost in an endless loop of worrying that other parents assume we are judging them. We cannot feed freely within a culture of scrutiny and enforced self-doubt.

In *The Bearded Lady* (1631), Spanish artist Jusepe de Ribera depicts a woman with a breast exposed, nursing her infant. Disappearing into the shadows behind is her husband, a ghostly presence within this deep chiaroscuro, wearing a worried frown and clasped hands. The woman is Magdalena Ventura, and she gazes at the viewer, confidently – defiantly – as if challenging us to recoil from her full, dark beard. Her facial hair is not the only marker of stereotypical masculinity; her hands are large and strong, her brow heavy and deeply lined, with a receding hairline. Ventura lived in Abruzzi and, according to the stone stele on the right of the canvas, she had three children before her thick beard appeared, in her late thirties. She became famous, a 'great wonder of nature', so much so that the Viceroy of Naples commissioned Ribera to paint her portrait. While her appearance would have earned her a living as a 'freak show', Ribera treats her with dignity. She looks us directly in the eye; there is no downward tilt of the chin, no turning away from her body. Her husband's concerned expression reveals the uncertain, and perhaps troubling, realities of their daily lives.

An interest in hirsute women was not unusual during this period, but what makes this painting unique is the presence of an infant and the suggestion of lactation. Her rounded, exposed breast reveals her femininity, redolent of the impossibly high, rounded breasts given to the *Madonna lactans* and therefore a visual trope seventeenth-century viewers would be familiar with. Her hands cradle this baby, whose lips brush but do not latch on to Ventura's very visible nipple. It's not clear if the baby is a symbolic addition to the painting, or whether Ventura had recently given birth. What is clear is that the baby at the breast – in this context – is a sign of Ventura's womanhood. Despite the dignity the painter gives her, she would have been regarded as an oddity rather than evidence of unstable gender binaries. However, centuries on, we can look at Ventura anew. Lactating bodies are all unique; none are disgusting. And yet.

Now, our icons are not Holy Mothers suckling divine babies. The average person sees between 6,000 and 10,000 adverts a day, a staggering amount of visual data; but very few will feature a woman breastfeeding or expressing breast milk with her hand. This unfamiliarity with the mechanics of breastfeeding may explain why one morning I opened Twitter to find a screenshot from my friend with the message 'have you seen this?'. I'd not seen this particular Facebook post, but its sentiment was not original and nor did it especially surprise me. The anonymised poster had written: 'I think it's pretty gross people breastfeed. It's not milk, it's bodily fluids. Might as well feed your little one your pee. We have bottles and formula ... that's meant to feed your baby. Stop giving your bodily fluid a classy name by calling it milk. IT'S NOT MILK. MILK COMES FROM COWS.' The post concluded with the words: 'Idiots everywhere'.

I've heard this before. About new mothers who refuse to breastfeed because it is 'dirty' or teenagers asking if a baby girl will catch 'lesbianism' from breastfeeding. Misinformation, lack of information, misogyny, histories of women's bodies being deemed messy, hysterical and unruly – a concatenation that results in breast milk being deemed disgusting. Because women's bodies in particular are viewed as messy and inconvenient. In *Inessential Women*, her 1988 book denouncing the exclusionary tactics employed by white, middle-class feminists, Elizabeth V. Spelman notes that '[w]hat might be called "somatophobia" (fear and disdain for the body) is part of a centuries-long tradition in Western culture'. More recently, Quill Rebecca Kukla, Professor of Philosophy at the Kennedy Institute of Ethics, has noted that for many parents, a lack of private space within their home can be as much of a barrier to breastfeeding as fears of public nursing. They go on to say that these parents:

likely do not have the kinds of bodies that we imagine as appropriately inhabiting such domestic space and hence as appropriately able to nurse. For these reasons, they may well not experience their bodies as able to breastfeed decently at all. They may feel, with justification, that the call to breastfeed is not really applicable to them, or that it is, but that they have no safe and comfortable way to respond to this call. It is worth making the effort to imagine how alienating images [promoting breastfeeding] must be to many women whose homes and bodies look absolutely nothing like this.[11]

It is true that imagery surrounding breastfeeding is still largely white, feminine, slim, cis and able-bodied. It creates a narrative that certain bodies are breastfeeding bodies, while others are not. And now, fear and disdain towards the female body and its functions coexists with the commodification of female flesh – and no part causes so much confusion as the female breast. Depending on who it belongs to and what it is doing, the female breast can represent all kinds of things: the potent sexuality of a pert, firm breast, the bestial aspects of humanity in the lactating breast or, in the withered breasts of witches, sin, Eve's temptation and the fall of man.

Yet the cultural chaos of the new mother's body is nothing compared to the outrage in some sectors of society over *male* lactating bodies. In 2013, Trevor MacDonald came to international attention when his application to volunteer with his local La Leche League chapter was blocked due to his gender identity.[12] MacDonald is a transgender man from Canada and parent to two children. He transitioned in his early twenties and, despite having had chest surgery, found that he was able to feed his child, with the help of a supplementary feeding system, when he became a parent in his thirties. LLL blocked him from becoming a group leader because he identified as a father.[13] He campaigned to change LLL's policy and the organisation removed gendered language from their policies.[14]

MacDonald joined a team of researchers to undertake pioneering studies into transgender men and pregnancy, birth and infant-feeding, funded by the Canadian Institutes of Health Research.[15] Speaking with twenty-two trans-gender men from across the world, the researchers found that many had not discussed future infant-feeding with their surgeons prior to undergoing chest surgery. Several men cited a worry that expressing a possible interest in nursing their babies at a later stage in life may negatively impact their chances of being approved for surgery, fearing that surgeons cleaved to a binary view of gender; expressing a curiosity about whether chest surgery may impact future parenting choices was deemed too risky in case the idea of a transmasculine person wishing to be associated with 'fem-inine' activity such as pregnancy or nursing was viewed as unintelligible by healthcare professionals. Later, after giving birth, the levels of dysphoria the men experienced while lactating varied widely. Some felt it so acutely they were no longer able to chestfeed, while others reported no feelings of dysphoria at all.

Trevor MacDonald's story, accompanied by photos of a bearded man with his shirt open, nursing his child, made headlines across the world. But individuals who have stereotypically male characteristics but breastfeed are not new. Biologically male, and non-birthing female, bodies can both lactate. Cisgender men feeding babies are dotted throughout literature, from the Talmud to a baby nurs-ing from an Englishman aboard a ship in Tolstoy's *Anna Karenina*. In Louise Erdrich's novel *The Antelope Wife*, a nineteenth-century US cavalry soldier, Private Scranton Teodorous Roy, finds himself lost in the wilds with a small baby. Unable to find a way to soothe the crying infant, he holds her to his nipples and is amazed when, days later, he begins to lactate in response to her suckling. When the let-down finally comes he is surprised by the pleasurable sensations it brings. In Buchi Emecheta's novel *The Joys of Motherhood*, Nnu Ego feeds a baby born to her husband's second wife, giving the child her 'virgin breast' and feeling surprised that, after a while, she begins to produce milk.[16] Away from fiction, Sir Astley Cooper, the Victorian surgeon who we encountered in Chapter 1, recorded a 22-year-old soldier who, from the age of eighteen, experienced 'prickling sensations' in his breast tissue, which was later accompanied by milky discharge. When he was examined in hospital, jets of milk would stream from his nipples. Astley gives no detail as to why this may have occurred, although today scientists argue that it is unlikely a man would begin to lactate from nipple stimulation alone unless the hormone prolactin were involved. But this can happen; a neurobiological problem or medication can cause the pituitary gland in men to overproduce prolactin, which could result in milk production, known as galactorrhea. Starvation can also cause spontaneous lactation, as observed in survivors of Nazi concentration camps and Japanese POW camps.

But our cultural devotion to the maternal is matched by our discomfort with considering lactation beyond the confines of the cisgendered female, maternal body. In 2003, the New Zealand Ministry of Health ordered a poster designed to encourage businesses to support breastfeeding in the workplace to be withdrawn as it showed a male actor holding a baby to his chest.[17] The poster was created by a women's health action group with the aim of making it clear that breastfeeding is not simply a 'women's issue' by subverting the iconography of the Madonna and Child. Moreover, non-biological parents are able to induce lactation, and I cannot tell of the envy I felt reading about the lesbian couple where the birth mother and her wife both breastfed their child. There are possibilities that offer emancipatory potentials for us all. While I doubt I would have wanted to share breastfeeding my son – given my extraordinary possessiveness towards his feeding – broadening our conceptual horizons may have taken some of the pressure off me too.

To achieve this, we need a subversion of breastfeeding iconography, to reinscribe the plurality of ways to be a nursing parent, and how that connects us to our own bodies and to society more broadly. As photographer Catherine Opie says, 'My nursing self-portrait is like the Madonna and Child, but at the same time, you see a forty-year-old lesbian with tattoos who had a baby. In a certain way, you can take the motif and push it to another place, so it has another iconography to it.'[18] The third instalment in a trilogy of self-portraits, Opie's *Self-Portrait/Nursing* (2004) depicts the artist cradling her infant, who tugs at her breast as they feed. A decade earlier she made *Self-Portrait/Cutting* and *Self-Portrait/Pervert*; the former is of her back, with a freshly carved childlike image of a house, cloud and two skirt-wearing stick figures. In the latter, the artist is wearing a gimp mask, with the word 'pervert' bleeding across her bare chest. The scar of the ornately inscribed word is just visible in *Self-Portrait/Nursing*, in which the artist, now revealing her face, breastfeeds her son. The brocade used as a backdrop in each image references Renaissance portrait conventions, symbolic of wealth and status; Opie's refiguring points to the levels of social acceptability given to members of LGBTQ+ communities and individuals. Opie characterised the butch S/M scene of 1990s California as being as much about radical politics and community as it was erotics, all of which offered her new ways to relate to her body. One imagines parenthood offered Opie similar experiences of reconfiguring community, politics and embodied identity.

What this tangle of media furore, art and protests tells us is that breastfeeding is ensnared in shifting cultural norms, patriarchal surveillance and the societal policing of vulnerable bodies. It is particularly cruel that all of this happens when we are at our most vulnerable. I glance now at my Rubens postcard and notice that although Mars is turned towards lactating Venus, his eyes are glancing down and away. He is, mentally at least, elsewhere and I can't decide if it's an attempt to protect her modesty or if he's simply bored by the whole thing. In any case, his emotional absence is significant; it is an acknowledgment that breast-feeding is viewed as 'women's business', the kind of labour we must do for emotional fulfilment, in private, and un-affected by the rest of the world.

CHAPTER 12

Sensational Bodies

A confession: sometimes I was so 'touched out' by the constant physical contact that breastfeeding repulsed me, and I wanted to bat the baby away. Another confession: sometimes breastfeeding arouses sensual reactions that one woman described as a 'non-sexual orgasm'. As a physical, intersubjective experience, lactation can encompass pleasure, submission, pain, curiosity, wonder, angst and desire. Sometimes all within the same twenty-four hours.

During the latter half of my baby's first year, he awoke at least once an hour every night, and the easiest way for us to get back to sleep was to place him on my boob. I was so tired and spent my days feeling as if my bones were turning to ash. Yet exhausted as I was, our daytime feeds had become luxurious moments of mutual rest and connection. There were transcendent moments, now the abject humiliation of the immediate post-partum period was behind me. It was those night feeds that hit hard. For the first thirty seconds I felt deeply, physically repulsed by the whole process. Every muscle in me tensed as my resentment poured out of me, thickening the air in the room. Until eventually, sleep returned.

I suspect none of this will be surprising for any parent. Yet these are the kinds of feelings that friends tell me of

in whispers. The kinds of ideas that, after an hour of conversation that takes in the minutiae of birth, interviewees
will begin to unspool hesitantly. Indeed, discussion of breastfeeding in any terms other than nutrition or health of the
baby, or talking about feelings beyond the sentimental,
remains rare and a kind of taboo. Perhaps because of the
parallel I am about to make: as with sex, there will be times
when nursing is pleasurable and times when it repels. We
don't often speak of this in relation to lactation because –
over centuries – the maternal breast has been denuded of its
possibility for sexuality. Think back to a few centuries ago,
when motherhood in western Europe was about tenderness
and devotion. To think of breastfeeding as offering potential
for 'a sensuous, non-commodified experience of our bodies'
is something we have, culturally, been restricted in doing.[1]
A boundary has been constructed between the maternal and
the sexual, and both states of being have, in the twenty-first
century, become sanitised and smoothed and commodified.

This unofficial prohibition has also resulted in a paucity
of language to describe the multiplicity and complexity of
bodily and emotional sensation. I wonder if we have lost
language and if our understanding of intimacy has been
flattened out and worn away, and if all we are left with is
a confusion of any other pleasurable bodily act with sex.
How are we to articulate the complexity of the breastfeeding experience when we don't have the words for the wide
assortment of processes and emotions it can entail? This can
range from true joy and pleasure through to ambivalence
and sheer pain, all physical as well as mental. As a culture
we tend to avoid thinking about breastfeeding being on this
spectrum, preferring to assume it is a largely pleasant and
tender neutrality that evokes enough motherly sacrifice and
infant satisfaction without edging into difficult territory. Yet
some voices do emerge unstifled. Poet Alicia Suskin Ostriker

writes of the pleasures but also shares those pains: 'she wants to kick – get off me, parasite. To kill it. To go mad'.[2]

Equally, parents who admit to sensual enjoyment of breast-feeding tell me of feelings of confusion within themselves, and expressions of judgement from others. A contented, sentimental mother is fine; a mother who enjoys the sensuous bodily feelings of breastfeeding is viewed with distaste, if not outright horror. It is thought that just under half of women will experience pleasurable sensations, which they may liken to sexual arousal, while breastfeeding. It's crucial to state that the physiological response to breastfeeding is a bodily response and completely normal. Breastfeeding provokes the nervous system and hormonal responses, and is a whole-body experience. Feelings of sexual arousal are simply involuntary bodily responses, usually to the flow of oxytocin or the physical stimulation of the nipple. But as it is not spoken about, women are less prepared to experience this kind of reaction, and can be unsure of where, if anywhere, is a safe space to discuss it. Suskin Ostriker writes of 'the erotic pleasure of nursing', noting that she has never seen mention of this kind of experience before despite pleasure surely being an important evolutionary response. She goes on, 'Why are mothers always represented sentimentally, as having some sort of altruistically self-sacrificing "maternal" feelings, as if they did not enjoy themselves? Is it so horrible if we enjoy ourselves: another love that dare not tell its name?'[3] Yet still we talk about the pleasures and pains of breastfeeding in constrained terms. In telling our stories, we often describe a delicate balance of enjoyment, but not too much, annoyance but not absolute revulsion. Parents I spoke to, like the eye-rolling woman from the last chapter, revealed that they tended to deploy a theatrical exasperation in front of family and friends, which concealed their true, complicated feelings about breastfeeding. Culturally we are so unused to seeing lactation, except when it is cultivated into an image deemed appropriate for public consumption. You can probably picture the kind of image I mean. You will have seen it on a poster in a clinic waiting room: a woman with just a touch of breast tissue exposed, gazing lovingly at the small baby in her arms. Overall, there is an absence of acknowledgement not just of pleasure or pain, but of sensuality in all its facets.

Culturally, there is often an assumption that anyone who chooses to breastfeed their children beyond their first or second birthday is doing so for selfish reasons, to satisfy their own emotional needs. The whole thing is shrouded in such darkness and fear over women's bodies. It is so pervasive that one woman I spoke to told me that, on finding out she was still breastfeeding her one-year-old, her paediatrician told her that it was 'disgusting', especially given the alternatives available, and that she was only doing it for her own 'pleasure'. In fact, nursing was irrelevant to the doctor's appointment, the woman had made no reference to how she felt about it, and the comments came entirely from the doctor's set of assumptions.

To understand the separation between the maternal and the sexual in the West, we need to consider the ways that female pleasure and motherhood have been conceptualised historically. In Elizabethan England, the female orgasm had been viewed as a necessary component to conception, an idea rooted in Hippocrates' notion of fertilisation requiring 'two seeds'. Female pleasure was therefore important, and this consideration of sensual experience extended to breastfeeding. Often these descriptions of the pleasures tip into the erotic. The sixteenth-century surgeon Ambroise Paré, who served four French kings, was unabashedly explicit: 'as the breast is tickled, the womb is aroused and feels a pleasurable titillation, since that little tip of the breast is very sensitive because of the nerves that end there'.[4] Midwife Martha Mears wrote in the 1790s that 'the act itself is attended with a sweet thrilling, and delightful sensations'.[5] In Thomas Stretzer's 1740 erotic tome, *A New Description of Merryland Containing A Topographical, Geographical, and Natural History of That Country*, he describes the female body as a terrain to explore; the book was so popular that between 1740 and 1742 it ran to ten editions. In this sexual bodily map-making, lactating breasts were landscapes undifferentiated from non-lactating: 'There are two other pleasant little Mountains called BBY, which tho' at some distance from MERRYLAND, have great Affinity with that Country. These little Mountains are exactly alike [. . .] on the Top of each is a fine foundation, that yields a very wholesome Liquor much esteemed, especially by the younger sort of People.'[6]

Yet despite this, the long-standing belief across western Europe that milk was formed from blood also meant a proscription on sexual intercourse in the post-partum period, given that sex 'troubleth the blood, and so in consequence the milk'.[7] Male sexual privilege was a prime reason for the popularity of wet-nursing in early modern Europe, allowing women to fulfil another strictly gendered role: sexually available, fertile and attractive wife. This is illustrated in a 1599 painting of Henri IV's advisor, mistress and confidante, Gabrielle d'Estrées, who sits upright in the bath, skin porcelain, breasts youthful and compact. Behind her a wet nurse feeds the baby, her breasts full, face rugged. Here is the maternal breast for the child, and the sexual breast for erotic display. Both breasts are available for consumption, but 'neither is owned by the woman herself'.[8]

As wet-nursing was discouraged and women were encouraged to nurse their own babies, the pleasurable aspects

of breastfeeding, for the mother, were more keenly emphasised. Addressing both parents in his essay on childrearing,
James Nelson, an eighteenth-century London apothecary
notes that: 'A man cannot be conversant with life and not
see that many a sensible woman, many a tender mother,
has her heart yearning to suckle her child, and is prevented
by the misplaced authority of her husband.'[9] In his view, it
was husbands who prevented their wives from nursing in
order to satisfy their own sexual interests in their wives'
breasts.[10] Nelson encouraged men to refrain from using
their male authority to prevent breastfeeding, as doing so
was to overturn both 'nature and reason'. Moreover, Nelson
gives attention to the pleasurable aspects of nursing which
may compensate a mother's 'anxiety and fatigue'. He writes:

> All mothers who have experienced it, whose minds are
> tempered with natural affection, assure us, that there is
> an inexpressible pleasure in giving suck, which none but
> mothers know; for besides the sensation itself is said to
> be mighty pleasing; to behold the innocence, the cun-
> ning, the tricks, and the various whims of a child; to
> observe likewise the early sentiments they discover; must
> doubtless give a pleasure which no words can describe.[11]

By this time, male medical writers were well aware of the
connection between nipple and clitoris, which was used to
explain why some women experienced agreeable sensations in regions other than the breasts while nursing. Yet,
pleasurable aspects of breastfeeding were largely deployed
in cultivating an image of a virtuous mother, while at the
same time effacing the messiness or orgasmic potential
of the reproductive body. By the nineteenth century, any
pleasurable aspect of breastfeeding had morphed into an
idealised and sentimental vision of motherhood. Maternal

nursing was now considered to be part of 'natural' motherhood. As one women's magazine from the 1840s wrote, the mother who nurses her child 'is conscious of a new principle of delight, physically and morally. The turbulence of love is past, and she has now that tranquil enjoyment best adapted to her health and her moral and intellectual growth.'[12] In addition, a woman's pleasure was no longer believed to be biologically required for reproduction. Attitudes towards women's desire became refashioned and constrained as this separation of reproduction and female pleasure contributed towards the cleaving of the maternal and the sexual: women were viewed as 'nurturing rather than desiring, as supportive rather than appetitive'.[13] By the end of the nineteenth century, female pleasure had become so sidelined that male doctors in France were specifically condemning and pathologising women who derived any pleasure from breastfeeding, describing women who did as suffering from mastomania.[14]

Maternity and romantic spousal love became the markers of a good mother. Mothers were to be modest and restrained and, crucially, they were not to appear to enjoy the base pleasures of the flesh, although many surely did. As motherhood was valorised, the maternal functions of the female body were emphasised, to the exclusion of any sexual function. In this scenario breastfeeding is effortless, not messy, not painful or taxing. The desexualisation of the pregnant and then nursing body was also a means to disempower women. This dynamic of child, mother and father locked in an eros of breastfeeding wasn't about female sexual liberation, but instead promoted the ideal of a natural and instinctual mother, who takes pleasure in breastfeeding. Furthermore, the separation of the maternal and the sexual meant that women's sexual gratification could only be granted by a man. As Iris Marion Young has noted, sexual pleasure from motherhood means the mother/child dyad becomes a closed circuit, meaning the man could become 'dispensable': 'patriarchy depends on the border between motherhood and sexuality. In our lives and desires it keeps women divided from themselves [. . .] the separation [. . .] seems to ensure her dependence on a man for pleasure'.[15]

If it took nearly a century for a women-centred interpretation of the Woman of Willendorf, then maybe it isn't surprising that three decades on, the idea of the statue being a self-portrait has yet to fully seep into our collective unconscious of what is possible. The theories that these voluptuous statues served a fertility or aphrodisiac function existed without reference to the possibility of them also being representative of a post-partum body. This either/or approach makes little sense in reality. Surely a good fertility fetish – if that is what the Woman of Willendorf was – is one that has successfully gestated, birthed and fed a baby? Is this an effect of a cultural framework still tinged with virginal Christian ideas of fertility without sex, of the potential before consummation? How could I integrate breastfeeding into my whole self? Could I ever imagine reclining naked on the bed, a baby at my breast, while my partner embraces me in a deep, passionate kiss? I saw this scene in an etching once, though I've not managed to find it since, and it was so troubling to me. Was it the conflating of the maternal body and the sexual body, both layered over each other so they coexisted in the same moment in time?

Sexual breasts are not supposed to be wet. They are not supposed to leak in response to anything other than the baby, or the thought of the baby. Keep your bra on if you are having sex, lest you leak, so the advice goes. As I delve into thinking about the breast as nourishing and the breast as erotic, I enter a Freudian dream where the satisfied milk-drunk baby anticipates the post-coital repose. Freud himself wrote that 'love and hunger' meet at the breast, but his interest in breastfeeding was largely confined to the role it played in the early psychosexual development of the infant. Iris Marion Young writes: 'breasts are a scandal because they shatter the border between motherhood and sexuality. Nipples are taboo because they are, quite literally, physically, functionally undecidable in the split between motherhood and sexuality.'[16] There is now a cultural amnesia about the breasts' lactating function.

I can't look at images of Mary across Western art history without thinking about her own sexuality. In many cases, although not all, motherhood and sex are inseparable. Isis reassembles her dismembered husband, fashioning him a new penis, so they can fully reunite and conceive a child. This is an act that, if things align, will set off a hormonal chain that culminates in lactation. But in a strictly binary sense, Mary emphasises the sexless, functional, maternal breast. It is Eve, clutching the apple that would transform her animal nakedness into shameful nudity, who presents the erotic and arousing breast. Pictured during her temptation and fall, Eve is not yet a mother, which makes her naked flesh scandalous. For many women, raised in a culture of Wonderbras and Page Three and online pornography, crossing this border and using their breasts to feed a baby is simply too uncomfortable. Or if the breasts are engaged in feeding a baby, they are 'off-limits' sexually. There is no in-between ground.

Questions of desire and pleasure can be swerved when the maternal body is viewed as a machine. As Fiona Giles has written, 'the virtues of breastfeeding represented by Christian iconography have been replaced by the equally reverential, scientific utility of breastfeeding; and both traditions are bound to the idea of the dutiful mother performing an act that verges on the sacrificial, whether constructed as spiritual or physiological'.[17] Discussions on breastfeeding usually fall under 'scientific' enquiry – talking about health benefits and nutrition, rather than the dazzling complexity of experiences, benefits and issues wrapped up in breastfeeding from the body. Think about the factory-style regulation of machine feeding, the weighing of babies and 'topping up' any deficit in production. The Industrial Revolution and modernity brought in new ideas of time and, with them, new ways of thinking about the body. The factory system fragmented craftsmanship into repetitive tasks at a machine and, so, the maternal body started to become thought of as a machine too, reducible to parts and tasks. The language used to describe maternal labour is often connected to the worlds of factories and production. Where is the idea of the body as a complex home? Where is the desire?

The cold, alabaster globe of the Virgin Mary's breast in Jean Fouquet's *The Virgin and Child Surrounded by Angels* (1450) challenges any binary of maternal and erotic. This detail from a diptych panel was painted for the Collegiate Church of Notre-Dame in Melun and is now housed in the Royal Museum of Fine Arts, Antwerp. It is a striking and vivid portrayal of Mary, cold and composed on her ornate throne, surrounded by fiery seraphim. Her left breast is completely exposed above her bodice and unobstructed by the naked baby perched on her lap, allowing the viewer to consume her nudity. Her porcelain skin, high hairline, and the absence of eyebrows was the height of fifteenth-century beauty. It is widely believed that the model for this Mary was Agnès Sorel, King Charles VII's official mistress and a woman who scandalised the French court by revealing more boob than was deemed appropriate. In 1445, the archbishop of Rheims, Jean Juvénal des Ursins, wrote to the chancellor of France – also his brother – to ask him to advise the king to end inappropriate fashions in the court. In his letter, the archbishop referred specifically to 'front openings through which one can see the teats, nipples, and breasts of women'. The decision to paint Sorel as the Virgin Mary with such a boldly exposed breast was an audacious one. The artifice of Mary's breasts in Fouquet's painting – likely deliberate – is artfully mocked by American artist Cindy Sherman (born 1954). The majority of Sherman's work consists of photographic self-portraits of the artist assuming different identities, playing with stereotypes of identity. In *Untitled #216* (1989), Sherman mimics the Nursing Madonna genre. The artist has downcast eyes, a blue shawl and a newborn cradled in her arm. Her bodice is open, revealing a spherical and quite obviously fake breast crudely stuck to her chest. The breast looks as if it may drop to the floor at any moment, being so divorced from Mary herself. This is not something exclusive to Fouquet, and many medieval painters placed the breasts in an unrealistically high position. But this wasn't due to their lack of knowledge of the female body. Instead, it was a gesture to the 'otherness' of Mary's lactation, which distinguished her from mortal women. After all, if her body leaked milk like other mothers' bodies leak milk then did she too bleed from her vagina? And if she bled from her vagina once a month, then could she be deemed to be without original sin? Therefore, the breast had to appear as an appendage at a remove from Mary herself.

Sherman further probes the portrayal of lactation in *Madonna lactans* art with two further images in this series. *Untitled #225* (1990) is a similar photographic pastiche of Renaissance tropes, but here Sherman includes the striking detail of a lactating (fake) breast, a drop of milk hanging delicately from the nipple. It is a striking homage to Sandro Botticelli, the Florentine painter responsible for several images of the Nursing Madonna, including *The Virgin*

and Child with Three Angels (Madonna del Padiglione)
(1493), in which Mary holds her breast and spurts milk
towards Christ. Sherman plays not only with the taboo of
bastardising religious motifs, but also the double taboo of
public lactation and the tightrope artists have walked when
representing divinity and titillation. It is also a reminder
that breast milk has not always been taboo or a reviled
substance in western Europe. Here is Botticelli, brush in
hand, delicately painting the 'white ink' across the canvas,
from the nipple to the mouth of Christ. Sherman's work is
also a stark reminder that most of the canonical examples
of the Nursing Madonna genre from the late medieval and
Renaissance periods were painted by men, all of whom
were looking at mothering from the outside in, like St Luke
with his stylus and paper. Perhaps this explains the notable
absence of Mary's maternal satisfaction or any sense of freedom and pleasure in her own body and that of her naked,
squishy baby.

I look at image after image and wonder, where is female
pleasure in all of this? What even *is* pleasure in this context?
Adrienne Rich wrote that nursing can be a sexual, erotic
act, a 'physically delicious, elementally soothing experience,
filled with a tender sensuality'.[18] I think back to the Woman
of Willendorf; she is full and ripe and motherly and sexual.
As if all the things our culture tells us are mutually exclusive
are combined within her as a powerful force, embodied in
that tiny statue.

One exception to all this maternal restraint and constraint
is Artemisia Gentileschi's *Madonna and Child*, painted in
1610, which offers an intimacy so clearly absent from many
other examples of the genre. Mary sits on a simple wooden
chair in an otherwise plain room. There are no cherubs or
saints interrupting the scene. The only clue that this is a
holy family comes from the hint of halo above each of their

heads. Mary is relaxed, her legs splayed to accommodate the infant reclining in her lap. Two fingers encircle her areola as she shapes the breast to meet the mouth of her distractible toddler. The boy reaches up to caress her face with his chubby hand, and he gazes at her with such gentle and serious love. Mary has closed her eyes in a state of contented bliss, relishing her baby's curious touch. There is something homely, down-to-earth and relatable here, even in the hint of exhaustion I detect in Mary's pose, the slight wilt in her composure. I recognise this paradoxical desire: wanting this moment to never end, but also desperate for the baby to hurry up and feed so everyone can go to bed.

The sensitivity to the subject matter is testament to Gentileschi's talent as an artist and observer. She was about twenty years old when she completed this painting and not yet a mother, and so was still an observer of the maternal experience. This reminds us that not only those with direct experience of motherhood are able to accurately render the experience, and not only because mothering can take so many different forms. Who can say why exactly Gentileschi was able to give such an accurate portrayal? Her father, Orazio, a contemporary of Caravaggio, painted his own versions, which are similarly earthy yet lack the palpable sense of oxytocin. His Mary holds her hand at an awkward angle behind the baby, who arches his back, as if she wants to avoid cradling him. Her other hand hoists her breast up into her neck. It is his daughter, Artemisia, who captures the paradoxical reality of lactation rendered in human-divine form. Here is the exhaustion of extended breastfeeding, all obliterated in one tender gesture from her child. Mary's body is noticeably not objectified in this scene, despite the nipple peeping out from between her fingers. The fleshy sensuousness of the image excludes the male gaze; there is no room here for phallic desire. It is in Gentileschi's

Madonna that I find Mary mothering and where I find a representation of my own eventual mothering reflected back at me.

Elsewhere, we tend to see lactation and sexuality through a lens of male heterosexuality. It is Jerry Hall, wearing a fur coat and heels, reclining in a plush chair while breast-feeding her son. The photograph, taken by Annie Leibovitz in 1999 and which appeared on the cover of *Vanity Fair*, is all red and gold, flesh tones and glossy blond hair. Or David LaChapelle's 1996 *Milk Maidens*, a cartoon-kitsch photograph of a lingerie-clad woman squirting breast milk into a bowl of cornflakes. Her back is arched, her hand sliding down to her groin, head thrown back and mouth wide open. It feels porny. While lactation porn and play is not in itself an issue, I do wonder what a maternal erotic that omits the male gaze might look like.

Just as breast milk was rendered in white paint across Renaissance canvases, so now it appears as a medium in its own right. In 2007 Jennifer West produced a short video work, using frozen breast milk and titled *My Milk Is Your Shit/Nirvana Alchemy Film 2,* where the milk plays on the surface of the 25mm film. This camera-less work was described in *Frieze* magazine by Joanna Kleinberg as 'a wild blend of synaesthetic experience wherein the substances of life literally and figuratively colour the film'.[19] But the milk isn't actually visible in the work. Instead, it forms part of the process, indistinguishable from the urine, perfume or pickle juice also present. The audience isn't confronted with the substance itself, simply the after-effect of bodily fluids.

Yet there are artists making lactation visible and exploring the multifaceted sensuality of breastfeeding. In 1998, the Los Angeles-based group M.A.M.A. (Mother Artists Making Art) made milk visible. The collective, comprising artists Lisa Mann, Athena Kanaris, Karen Schwenkmeyer, Deborah Oliver and Lisa Schoyer, came together via parenthood; two members met in a breastfeeding support group. This foundation underscores the desire not only for community, but also for one that enables a validation of their maternal experiences. On a practical level, new responsibilities meant they feared not being able to make work individually; but together they could push one another. At the time, the collective wrote about: 'support[ing] each other in salvaging, theorizing and representing through artworks, our experience of being mothers, especially in teasing out those experiences which are invisible or taboo in terms of the norms (for example the sensual possibilities of pregnancy, breastfeeding and the relation of mother and child, are taboo in this culture.)'.[20]

They now look back and concede that the collective was also a political action, not only in their work but also in the very act of organising as a group. And it was in their work *Milkstained* that lactation was made corporeally manifest on a public stage, exploring the sensations of breastfeeding. It was a multi-sensory performance to a small audience at the Electronic Café International in Santa Monica, also live-streamed on the internet. The performance began with a naked woman lying on a white fabric pedestal, her back to the audience, white cloth draped over her buttocks and thighs. The pose is familiar, the curves of the back and waist and hips, the languid movement of the falling cloth that reveals as much as it conceals. This is very much a classical female nude. Yet it is soon interrupted by white liquid pouring down her back, flowing onto the white cloth, damp patches blossoming. More women join the stage, some expressing milk by hand, others pouring milk into a fountain of cocktail glasses.

The performance also included spoken word, the sounds

of a baby feeding, and the unmistakable whirr of an electric breast pump expressing milk. At the end, the audience was invited to taste the fresh milk. *Milkstained* underscored the disorder of the maternal body, the 'uncontrollable, hysterical fluids – blood, milk, emotions, tears'.[21] The performance rendered the messiness of motherhood visible, the noises audible.[22] And, in forcing the audience to confront their own taboos, also challenged the viewer to think about how this messiness can be sensual, and pleasing. There's a radical honesty in the work that sends me reeling, a heady mix of vulnerability and empowerment that rushed me back to those early, visceral goddesses.

The small audiences at M.A.M.A.'s performances were self-selecting participants. But the collective also created work for the unwitting member of the public to discover. In *California Civil Code Section 43* (1998), M.A.M.A. referenced the state law that protects a woman's right to breastfeed in any location, public or private. A wooden box measuring 18 inches square was placed on a public bench in a retail area in Pasadena. A large X, like a ballot, was painted on the front of the box, while its lid and sides were decorated with cartoon animals suckling their offspring, like a child's alphabet block, with the X also conjuring ideas of consent and censorship. A speaker concealed inside played the sounds of a baby's incessant cry. When intrigued passers-by opened the box they found a monitor showing videos of women breastfeeding, each shot from the perspective of the mother looking down at her baby. A voiceover recounted women's experiences of breastfeeding and their complicated attitudes towards their bodies, the changes that they have undergone as their body becomes an 'object of desire – a simultaneous source of sexuality and nourishment'.[23]

The artists kindly shared with me the footage from inside

that box, the same footage that had been shown on screens during the *Milkstained* performance. Watching it at home, alone, I felt as if I was intruding on profoundly intimate moments. The closeness and obvious, deep pleasure experienced by the child, if not also the mother, is an extraordinary expression of deep love. The babies moan and sigh, the sounds of wet lips on skin, kissing noises, and a long deep 'mmmmhhh, mmmmhh'. A chubby hand releases a nipple from a white lace bra – boo! – with an intense interest. A woman hums a lullaby as a child fiddles with their own anatomy while feeding. It is beautiful, as all boundaries that we navigate between our sensuous selves are broken down.

This was the first time I had seen the realities of my own breastfeeding experience reflected back at me in ways that were mundane and at the same time intensely transcendent.

Today, remembering that little box, Lisa Mann, Karen Schwenkmeyer and Lisa Schoyer recall that teenage girls looking into it tended towards curiosity, while boys were overtly disgusted. These adolescent boys made it clear that breasts were sexual and belonged to them. How can we reclaim ourselves within a heteronormative patriarchy, when a body can be fragmented into parts, parts that are often thought of as detached from the self? No wonder we talk of our lactating breasts as 'not feeling like mine' or 'no longer belonging to me'. We can lay the blame for these feelings on the corporeal, relentless task of caregiving an infant. But equal responsibility lies with the historical prioritisation of male sexuality and convenience, at times at the expense of the well-being of parents and babies. Heteronormativity and the idea of the nuclear family has deleterious effects on everyone. The 'cultural amnesia' that we have around nursing, thanks to changes since industrialisation and the marketing of formula, as well as the associated loss of communal bonds, means that breastfeeding can be a lonely experience; and all the more so if experiences, desires and sensations appear to be outside of normative boundaries. To overcome this we need collaboration and, like the M.A.M.A. group, to reclaim our autonomy, find support and connection, and develop safe spaces to revel in the entirety of our being.

CHAPTER 13

Milk Ecologies

Milk blooms from the corners of his mouth, overflowing as he mechanically sucks. The first night that he sleeps for longer than usual, I wake up soaked and confused, trapped under two hard rocks. I watch milk collect, drop by painful drop, in my manual breast pump. Pour it into little ziplock bags to be frozen, open the fridge to see little bottles of it stored in the back, next to the butter and cheese. Later, at work, expressing in the toilets at lunchtime, I chug the warm milk rather than deposit it down the drain. If I'm going to all the trouble to make it, I may as well recycle as much of that energy as possible. My milk tastes watery and sweet, like nothing I've ever had before but overwhelmingly familiar. Over time, I did a lot of looking at my own breast milk, smelling it, tasting it. Not with any degree of real contemplation. It was just there. A fact of me. A fact of life.

Would you drink breast milk? Did you try your own? Would you use it in tea if you couldn't be bothered to nip to the corner shop? Would you drink someone else's milk? Would you savour the flavours? What kind of interconnectedness would that open up? Did you realise your mother's milk was part of a wider ecology? That we are inextricably connected?

The idea for hosting a breastmilk tasting session came

to artist Jess Dobkin while she was pregnant. She had long been interested in challenging boundaries and exploring queer identities in her performance work, so the idea of seeking out milk donors and offering audiences the chance to try different milks appealed. It was an idea born of curiosity and of wondering how to unite her burgeoning life as a parent with her work as an artist. As Canada emerged from lockdown, she spoke to me from the office of the gallery where she was busy installing her latest work. Despite it being sixteen years since she conceived of the idea, her enthusiasm and delight in talking about milk hasn't waned: 'My gosh, today I'm gonna say sacred, but it's kind of this boundless substance where it's like, a bodily fluid, and it's a food and we produce it from our bodies, and it changes over time.' A performance where she shared her milk would be a chance to explore this boundlessness, through an act of hospitality where she and others might donate milk. Yet after giving birth, Dobkin experienced a slew of familiar issues with breastfeeding. This, coupled with a lack of meaningful support, meant she was left unable to continue nursing her daughter and with a feeling of, as she described it at the time, 'not measuring up'. The project she had planned during pregnancy shifted; it had never in any case been meant solely as a promotion of breastfeeding over all other methods, but the final performances, titled *Lactation Station*, became imbricated into a longer artistic and personal journey of exploration and healing.

The first *Lactation Station* 'happening' took place in Toronto in 2006, as part of a broader programme of performance art around the theme of 'taste'. Dobkin was pleasantly surprised by how generous and trusting people were in donating milk, which was pasteurised and culture-tested in line with health regulations. Bar spaces were installed in the gallery and small groups were invited to try two milk samples each and reflect on the taste. Often remembered now simply for this aspect, *Lactation Station* also involved in-depth interviews with milk donors, whose stories played on video in the gallery during the tastings. Dobkin felt a great responsibility towards the donors, and her care for them was meticulous. She also placed a degree of trust in the audiences, hoping they would be respectful and avoid the shock value tropes common in headline reporting of the events; she was aware that the set-up was an invitation to engage in a taboo activity. This meant she placed extra emphasis on designing the events to give a sense of order and familiarity, with a maître'd and milk menus. The gallery context was less about delineating the experience as 'art' and more about the kind of environment offered by a white cube space, with its clean walls conveying a sense of hygiene. The nice space and good service plays with the paradoxical position of milk as a revered substance, while also being something that needs to be made 'safe'.

Lactation Station has been staged three times, in 2006, 2012 and 2016, and Dobkin sensed the cultural shifts that were taking place over this period, largely ascribable to the rise of social media and the potential for online connectivity, support and conversation. In organising and hosting, the artist reciprocated the enormous generosity and trust donors and samplers had placed in her. The events unfolded as conversations, playing with the dynamic of Dobkin as host and sommelier, the audience of tasters and non-tasters, and the donors. But the focus was ultimately the milk itself, each one differentiated by a unique name and backstory, based on interviews the donors had given to Dobkin. As people drank from tiny plastic glasses of 'Sweet Fall Harvest' and 'Passion's Legacy', the artist advised them on the woman's diet at time of expressing, the age of their child, and details of the woman's experiences with breastfeeding.

Breast milk was made specific, a reminder of its universality but also a reminder of an ethics and duty of care to parents, the producers of the milk that is so highly prized.

It means something, to read a food and drink critic consider breast milk:

> Breast milk has a silky mouthfeel [. . .] as for aftertaste? That varied the most. [. . .] The first sample I tried was nutty, slightly sweet and had the consistency and mouthfeel of watered-down soy milk. It was called Life Force Elixir, and felt like it. [. . .] The second, nicknamed Temple of the Goddess [. . .] had a surprisingly angry aftertaste that several on the tasting panel agreed shot directly up one's nose and stayed there. Dobkin advised the mother who supplied it had consumed highly spiced food around that time.[1]

In all the material I have read on milk, this is one of the few descriptions that give clarity and attention to the substance itself. *Lactation Station* attempted to isolate the milk from the donor, yet in the tasting it was impossible to remove the trace of the maker. While the donor was evoked through the naming of the milk, the conversations Dobkin facilitated, and their testimony on the gallery walls, their actual labour involved in the lactation was private. Audience members were not privy to the processes involved and instead the final product was served at a bodily remove from the means of its production. How different would the experience be, for donors and tasters, if they had heard the rhythmic whirr of a breast pump, saw the nipple distend and stretch and the milk spray into the bottle? It is a reminder that for all the glamorous photoshoots with women wearing breast pumps, it is an activity that is often hidden from view, so animalistic and mechanistic that we do not even contemplate doing it in a public place. Dobkin plays with this idea too, allowing the promotional posters for *Lactation Station* to be ribald and humorous as a counterpoint to the care and respect of the event itself. It's a striking photograph, of the topless artist manipulating her own breast to jet a substantial arc of breast milk into a wine glass. It is wildly unrealistic, not in quantity of milk but in the obedience of the milk in hitting its target. It looks adult and porny, even down to the wine glasses, and it reminds us that the public health authorities in Toronto instructed the gallery to place highly visible signs around the space stating that it was forbidden for minors to sample the breast milk. Milk was for adults only.

Lactation is often thought of as a process or practice, and rarely do we think about the product itself – milk – outside of child-rearing contexts. In directing our attention to the product Dobkin forces us to consider its origins, challenging capitalist and consumer tropes with ideas of gift and hospitality. Under what conditions was the milk produced? What processes are involved? What value do we place on the labour of lactation and how taboo do we really think the final product is? How does paid work intersect with the work of mothering? And what are the contours of the paradox where breast milk can be positioned as a commodity while the labour involved in producing it is not properly acknowledged or remunerated? Before I had a baby these questions seemed to me a little abstract, and remained so even after I gave birth, with my public health services and statutory maternity pay. This not only gave me the freedom to establish breastfeeding before returning to work, it also compensated me – in theory – for my maternal labour. Motherhood became my paid work. When I think about the terminology, they are all *doing* words: Breastfeeding. Giving suck. Nursing. Nourishing. Suckling. Giving milk. Lactating. Expressing. Pumping. Sterilising. Wet-nursing.

Bottle-feeding. Whichever way we do it, there is activity involved and a passage of time. *Our time*. (If I had thought about this in my early motherhood, I might have realised it is an activity that one can get better at, through practice). The idea of the 'naturalness' of breastfeeding often masks a lack of funding for mothers and support services.[2] If it is framed as a 'natural' and fulfilling role for women, then it is not deemed 'work' and, therefore, the burden and costs associated with breastfeeding fall on women. When women use substitutes for breastfeeding, they can be viewed as lazy and/or responsible for any negative health outcomes, rather than seen as making the best choices they can within their circumstances.

The baby mewls. I lift my shirt, he latches, and there I will sit for minutes, possibly hours, over and over again, day after day. Even between feeds, my body cannot rest. It is busy, converting the vast amount of food I'm now compelled to consume into milk. There are no breaks. My mum cuts up my lunch for me. I'm adept at using my left hand to eat it now. This is my maternal labour and I have timesheets to prove it; in the hospital, they tell me to record the time of each feed and note each nappy change. We dutifully do this on the back of an A4 photocopied leaflet about pelvic floor exercises. 12.04 a.m. L; 12.37 a.m. R, and so on. Later, when we get home from our second hospital visit, when I must breastfeed, express, bottle-feed, I find an app and scrabble to hit 'start feed' whenever my son latches. There are statistics and graphs, which I pore over but which never make me feel better.

What makes me feel better is when I tire of tracking feeds and nappies and sleep, when I tire of regime feeding and try to adapt to a new sense of time. My baby is seven weeks old and I've come to stay with my parents. I am frantic and lost. One afternoon my dad says, simply, 'There are about six reasons why a baby will cry: hunger, nappy, tiredness, boredom, temperature or overstimulation. Run through the checklist, then you'll realise sometimes they just cry because they need to cry. You'll learn to discern the differences in time.' My dad is the only person my baby will fall asleep with other than me and, occasionally, my partner. Even when he was small, I would watch his tiny body relax into my father's chest. I was rarely relaxed myself, perhaps because I was working. Sometimes I envied my son and longed to be small enough to bury into the wool and smoke smell and be held completely in my father's arms. I will always be a mother and I will always be a child.

The 1881 UK census was the first to classify housewives as unoccupied, an expression of the bureaucratic impact of the separation of work and motherhood. The fashioning of the family into a unit of consumption rather than production. It was brutal because working mothers could no longer juggle childcare and paid work. They were no longer free to pause work to attend to a hungry baby. The master of Dutch interiors, Quiringh van Brekelenkam, gives us an insight into what the relationship between mothering and paid work might have looked like. In *Interior of a Tailor's Shop*, painted around 1655–6, a tailor and his two assistants sit cross-legged on a table by the window, the only light source in the room. To the other side of the pictorial field a woman sits on a low stool to the left of the fire, nursing an infant. Presumably she is the tailor's wife and once the baby is satiated, she will pick up her bobbin pillow or pail and continue with her work – activities depicted in similar scenes by the same artist. Negotiating breastfeeding and other activities is also illustrated by a rare sixth-century bronze from Indonesia, an early example of a parent multitasking.

The bronze is just 25cm tall. A woman sits upright, her body forming a 90-degree right angle with the ground. She wears a calf-length skirt and her hair hangs in a long plait down the length of her spine. In her arms she cradles a small baby, who feeds from her left breast. Whoever made this sculpture was familiar with how babies feed; the infant's hand tweaks and fiddles with the woman's right nipple as they feed. The woman is also wearing a simple bead necklace and large hooped earrings. I wonder if the child tugs at these while nursing too? A loom rests on her extended legs, braced by her flexed feet. This scene is one of interruptions; she has paused her weaving to pick up the hungry baby. She cannot work the loom and hold her child at the same time. Soon she will place the baby down and resume her weaving, moving from one task to another. This sculpture offers a window into the everyday moments of a mother's life.

Shared nursing, also called allonursing, is found across cultures. Sometimes it is only used in extreme circumstances, such as in the event of the biological mother's death, serious illness or inability to produce milk. Elsewhere, women nurse babies when the mother must travel away from the family. The word for woman in one cultural group in the Andaman Islands in the Indian Ocean is 'milky breast' and, in this culture, if a mother has to leave her child, another woman will suckle her baby and will be deemed to be a 'good milky breast' for having done so.[3] In societies where shared feeding is common, social codes usually underpin the practice. For example, biological mothers like to know what the other nursing parents are eating, in case they have consumed taboo foods that could harm the baby. Elsewhere, it is usually women biologically related to the child who undertake the role, most commonly grandmothers. And if you are wondering if these postmenopausal grandmothers are still able to produce milk, several male anthropologists have reported asking the same question and getting a squirt of breast milk in reply.

Wet-nursing conventions also reveal ideas about kinship bonds. For example, the Quran forbids men from having sexual relationships with anyone with whom they have a milk relationship, which would be anyone from whom they nursed or who had shared a nurse with them. The idea of milk-mothers and milk-sisters ruled out marriage with any other children who were nursed by the same wet nurse, and marriage plans would be cancelled if a milk relationship was discovered – often based on the testimony of the wet nurse herself. The basis for this milk relationship comes from the ancient idea of milk being transformed blood from the womb, and blood confers kinship.[4] The milk relationships also had the additional benefits of extending kinship networks and familial alliances.

Histories of breast milk are complex and fraught, and reveal that the transfer of milk is about more than nutrition. Woven into sustenance are bodies and money, class and sex, morality and socialisation, all of which are culturally dependent. In the UK, there are many women who have nursed babies belonging to their friends or family and who have done so for a wide variety of reasons. But the extent to which the idea of wet-nursing has fallen out of public favour in twenty-first Britain is demonstrated by the fact that even in the midst of our own feeding struggles, it was never suggested that I might look into the milk of another woman. And despite knowing that milk banks existed, the thought of sourcing breast milk from elsewhere never occurred to me either.

CHAPTER 14

Wet-Nursing

Three rivulets of milk combine into two droplets, suspended above the parted lips of a baby. The yellow and white brushstrokes hold the moment in stasis and we are left to anticipate the flow of milk into the mouth, down the throat and then into the tiny tummy. The breast from which the milk flows has been dissected, the skin removed to reveal the tissues and webs of ducts and globules. Two drops of milk fall from the other, undissected breast, towards the infant's dress, where we must imagine they will bloom into white flowers stretching towards the delicate lace hem. Fat milky drops of rain fall from the brooding sky, whose heavy grey clouds contrast with the vivid verdant jungle backdrop. The woman's black hair frames a dark and haunting face. The infant has adult features, reminiscent of the homuncular Jesus found in medieval Madonna and Child paintings, where Jesus' balding hairline and old-man face symbolised his preternatural knowledge and wisdom. But this child is bored and listless. There is something unsettling about this version of the Madonna and Child.

Yet the baby's face is instantly recognisable. The thick, unbroken black brow and subtle shadow above lipstick-red lips indisputably identify this as being Frida Kahlo. It is a face that has now become so ubiquitous that Theresa May wore it on a bracelet at the 2017 Conservative Party Conference. (This commodification is perhaps ironic for a former member of the Mexican Communist Party, who changed her year of birth from 1907 to 1910 so that it coincided precisely with the Mexican Revolution). In *My Nurse and I* (1937), Kahlo's famous features appear in an uncanny juxtaposition with the bare-breasted woman whose own face is hidden beneath a black, stony mask.

Kahlo was the daughter of a German-Jewish migrant and his Mexican wife. As an infant, she was cared for by an indigenous wet nurse after her mother fell ill. One of Kahlo's biographers recounts the artist telling a friend, 'I was nursed by a nana whose breasts they washed every time I was going to suckle.'[1] While her father was an atheist, Kahlo's mother was a devout Catholic and tried to raise the children in the faith. Trips to church would have exposed Kahlo to plenty of representations of the Holy Mother; *My Nurse and I* takes its form from Mexican ex-voto paintings, Catholic offerings of thanks for salvation after an accident or an illness.

Kahlo was proud of her milky connection to Mexican indigeneity. The name of her wet nurse has been lost to history, but the painting of her reveals Kahlo's sustained political and artistic interest in pre-colonial Mexican culture and her own heritage. She and her husband, muralist Diego Riveria, were collectors of pre-Columbian artefacts, including masks; and, as one art historian has suggested, 'the nurse arguably becomes a symbol of the artist's own mestiza origin, but the relationship between the different elements is an uneasy one'.[2] The significance of women in early Mesoamerican culture has long been overlooked by scholars, but it is a culture where representations of motherhood abound.[3] The Metropolitan Museum of Art in New York holds a riveting example. Dating from between

100 BCE and 200 CE and found in a tomb in western Mexico, it is a terracotta sculpture of a woman nursing a baby, and also functions as a rattle. Kahlo was well versed in Mesoamerican and Aztec cultures and would have been familiar with their iconographies. Her Mother and Child composition in *My Nurse and I* melds the Catholic Madonna with the indigenous universal goddess, while the verdant background suggests a link to the Ceiba tree, whose trunk was believed to connect the underworld and the sky to the terrestrial plane. The Ceiba was also thought to nourish babies who had died with its pendulous fruits.[4] The baby's dress is reminiscent of a Catholic christening gown, while the woman's mask is like those used in Aztec ritual sacrifices.

The common story behind the painting is that Kahlo painted the woman wearing a mask because she could not remember her face or accurately portray her. Yet the masking of the nurse mirrors a different kind of masking of Kahlo's face. There is an ambivalence; we cannot begin to discern what emotions might lie beneath the wet nurse's mask. Similarly, Kahlo stares into the middle distance, her face blank and detached, her mouth not even touching the nurse's flesh. The power of Kahlo's oeuvre lies in her ability to represent fragmentations of subjectivity and marginalisation of self, by token of gender, ethnicity or political persuasion. Wet-nursing itself can represent fragmentation as well as union. At times, the practice of women feeding babies other than their own solidifies communities and strengthens bonds. At other times, it impacts marginalised groups and the autonomy of a woman over her own body.

Wet-nursing has been a transcultural practice, and industry, possibly for as long as mothers have been having babies. In the absence of formula, clean water or pasteurised milk, the milk of another human offers a reliable alternative to a biological mother's milk; shared breastfeeding would have originated with need before it became associated with ideas of choice and social status. *My Nurse and I* raises questions about milk, the work of the body that makes it and the bonds between those who share it. Moreover, it draws our attention to the gendered, racial and economic disparities that can underpin such arrangements.

In the *Republic*, Plato argued that babies should be housed in public nurseries and fed by wet nurses in order to strengthen their allegiance to the state. The closest the world has ever got to seeing this idea play out is in Paris, where rapid urbanisation and industrialisation led to whole wet-nursing industries. Wet-nursing had been a well-organised operation in France from the twelfth century onwards, but by the end of the eighteenth century, almost half the babies whose births were recorded in Paris were placed with rural wet nurses. A detailed survey by Lieutenant General Jean-Charles-Pierre Lenoir revealed that in 1780 only 3 per cent of Parisian babies were nursed by their own mothers. Another 3 per cent were fed at their home by a wet nurse. But most babies were sent to foundling hospitals or rural areas to be nursed by a stranger, with placements arranged by Le Bureau des Nourrices, an official institution founded in 1769. What that means is that roughly 10,000 babies were leaving the city – and their parents – each year.

This was happening while Rousseau was encouraging women to breastfeed their own babies for the moral good of the nation. While this shift in attitudes saw an increase in aristocratic women breastfeeding, urban middle- and working-class women still found breastfeeding and employment incompatible. Their economic and social conditions meant it was largely impossible for employed women to nurse their own babies. The slower economic development in the rural regions outside of Paris therefore produced 'the unique phenomenon of a vast, organised activity of peasant women nursing urban infants for pay.'[5] For example, in the small French city of Besançon, women found it more economical to work in the famous watch factories and pay a rural wet nurse.[6] Parents clearly wanted their children to gain the benefits of breast milk, but it simply wasn't viable for mothers to both work and breastfeed their own children.

Despite being a working parent well acquainted with balancing child-rearing and employment, I cannot fathom what this kind of system looked like – or what it felt like. Shared feeding, within close communities, resonates within me at a deep level. But a mass exodus of babies to be fed elsewhere seems incomprehensible, especially when viewed alongside the movements encouraging maternal nursing. The bind parents find themselves caught in and the mismatch between rhetoric and practical support is still depressingly familiar today. I search the archives of the Museums of Paris for depictions of what wet-nursing on this scale might have looked like. Or rather, to get a sense of how people wanted this phenomenon to be recorded. I find stacks of eighteenth-century prints, some showing well-dressed ladies in all their pomp handing babies over to plainly dressed women with ample bosoms. We get a sense of the scale and organisation involved from looking at prints of women touring Le Bureau des Nourrices, looking for suitable nurses for their children, aided by *meneurs*. These were the men who recruited women in the countryside, brought them to and from Paris, and arranged payments and updates between nurses and parents. There are prints of high-class couples visiting the house of the wet nurses, the delicate figures of eighteenth-century maternal mothers contrasting with the plump, sturdy wet nurses, suggesting a class-based aptitude for lactating: the middle-class women are far too dainty for such a task. Caricature sketches of doughy peasant women breastfeeding are common in the archives. On the one hand, rural women were viewed as hardy and perfectly suited to the tasks involved in raising infants. On the other hand, terrible stories circulated: wet nurses taking in too many charges to care for, weaning the baby too early, substituting a foundling for a baby who had died.

Paintings of this era tell of the emotional pain of leaving a child with a wet nurse. In Etienne Aubry's *Farewell to the Nurse (Les Adieux a la Nourrice)*, painted in 1777, a toddler squirms away from his well-dressed mother, desperate not to be separated from the arms of his nurse. The wet nurse's husband leans towards the infant, noticeably emotional, while the child's father stands apart and aloof. Cartoons lampooning not only paternal alienation but also the very fact of paternity abound too, as well-dressed men reach for furious babies in the arms of rosy-cheeked nurses. In one the man says to a hesitant child, 'Come and kiss you papa my dear,' while the nurse replies, 'Yesterday his mother came to see him with your moustachioed cousin, and he kissed her right away.'

Diderot wrote of Jean-Baptiste Greuze that his art is 'dramatic poetry that touches our feelings, instructs us, improves us and invites us to virtuous action'.[7] Greuze's 1765 work *The Beloved Mother,* one of the most popular paintings of the thirteen or so he displayed at the official art exhibition of the Académie des Beaux-Arts in Paris – known as The Salon – in that same year, depicts the blissful joy of parenthood. A mother reclines amid a sea of children, her upturned face tender yet strained; her husband is walking in, arms and smile wide, heart thrust forward with delight at returning to his family. Diderot again: 'he paints a sympathetic picture of the happiness and advantages deriving from domesticity; it announces to any man with soul and feelings: Maintain your family comfortably, make children with your wife, as many as you can, but only with her, and you can be sure of a happy home.'

On the other hand, *The Nursemaids*, his portrayal of rural wet nurses painted *c*.1765, about three years after the French-language publication of Rousseau's *Emile*, couldn't be more different. It depicts the potential destination for infants once they arrived in the countryside, and acts as a warning that supports Rousseau's text: children raised in such environments will become unruly and immoral adults. Two women sit in a dark interior, its contents in disarray on a dirty earthen floor, grey laundry strung out across the room. The scene invokes a claustrophobic dampness. A little light filters across the canvas, illuminating the worn face of the older nurse, a child asleep in her arms. A toddler buries her face in the bosom of a younger nurse – it's not clear if she is feeding or not. Four other toddlers litter the room, one playing with a dog, another boy holding a bird, another cowering behind the older children.

This tableau of grime contrasts sharply with scenes of the in-house nurses the wealthy could afford. In one print from the 1820s by Jean-Pierre Mallet, a young woman sits in an ornate room, her chair next to a table holding a gold platter. She is breastfeeding an infant, who lies across a pouffe reaching for her breast. The woman's eyes angle down, but her upper body tilts away from the baby so there is minimal contact between the two. Directly behind her a man leans against a large dresser, wearing a felt hat and cloak, casually watching us the viewer. His wife stands to the right, her body facing away. Yet she is looking over her right shoulder at us, her hand buried in the lush white satin folds of her dress. She is stiff, unemotional, awkward even. There is a palpable lack of warmth between any actors in the scene. Intimacy and emotion are left hanging in both scenes of rural squalor and urban pomp.

*

I learned about Saint Agatha from a painting by the seventeenth-century Spanish artist Francisco de Zurbarán, in which a young woman holds a pair of severed breasts on a plate. She holds the platter across her body, tilting it slightly towards the viewer as if proudly showing us a cake she has baked. Beyond a barely perceptible concave chest, what this painting does not make clear is this: those breasts are hers.

Painted as slovenly and neglectful, wet nurses were often vulnerable to exploitation and abuse, in Europe as well as in the colonies, where enslaved women were coerced into nursing white settlers' babies. Seldom is concern towards wet nurses found in the literature. In the nineteenth century, Sir Astley Cooper wrote of a patient who employed a wet nurse for her two children for a period of three years in total. While the children were healthy and strong, the nurse was so weakened 'as to be incapacitated from any useful labour'. The family who employed her showed mercy by 'keeping her, but no longer as an efficient servant'.[8] Bad-mouthing wet-nursing allowed companies and shareholders to profit from the sale of artificial formula. But what of these wet nurses?

Saint Agatha is believed to have been born in Sicily in the third century and to have decided, from an early age, to dedicate her life to God. Her vow of chastity didn't prevent the advances of the Roman prefect Quintianus, whom Agatha repeatedly repudiated. Quintianus, fragile of ego and unable to take rejection, eventually had her imprisoned. He hoped the threat of torture would be enough to break her resolve, but instead of submitting to his advances she prayed for courage. The authorities tortured her; she was stretched on a rack, whipped and burned. Eventually, when she still refused to capitulate, Quintianus ordered that her breasts be cut off with pincers. She was then sentenced to be burned at the stake but, after an earthquake, she was instead sent back to prison, where her wounds were healed by a vision of St Peter the Apostle.

There is a cruel specificity to her punishment. In her commitment to chastity and her rejection of marriage, the visual markers of her femininity are excised. In de Zurbarán's painting of her, not a trace of her torments is visible on her face. Instead, she raises her eyes wearily to the viewer, her delicate beauty offset by the blood-red robe that flows from the nape of her neck down to the ground. The removal of her breasts – a metaphor for the loss of agency over her own body – means that Saint Agatha is the patron saint of both breast cancer patients and wet nurses; categories of women who, arguably, have lost control of their breasts.

The beliefs and practices surrounding shared feeding are as specific as the ways communities were organised. Much can be gleaned about the practices of and status afforded to wet nurses from medical texts, legal codes, and contracts and receipts from wage payments, written on papyri. Unsurprisingly for a practice integral to the survival of infants, wet-nursing was sometimes codified with legal language, and there was status attached to nourishing elite infants. In Ancient Egypt, wet nurses were used for royal babies and these wet nurses' biological children were legally permitted to call themselves 'milk-kin' of the king. These nurses were represented in tomb paintings and referred to as the 'Royal Nurse', and women who nursed boys who went on to be king were sometimes given the title of 'One Who Nurtured the God'.[9] In socially stratified Ancient Greece, too, wet nurses were utilised by women of high socioeconomic status, which would often then 'rub off' on the wet nurse, even though the latter tended to be enslaved and lived in the child's home, which meant their diet, behaviour and sexual activity could be closely monitored. It was rare in Ancient Greece for a nurse to be characterised as neglectful and, in literary texts, they are portrayed as devoted. In written contracts, there is evidence of material concern extended to the wet nurse too: gifts of gold earrings, or annual feasts. Wet nurses tended to hold high positions in Southeast Asian cultures, too; in some Buddhist cultures in these regions, a wet nurse was a symbol of generosity, so much so that evidence shows that rulers left great wealth to their wet nurses to repay them the debt they believed they were owed.

The fact of status being afforded to a wet nurse gives a sense of a relationship between the wet nurse and her charge where it is not only milk being transmitted from the woman but also status transferred from the baby. Wet-nursing myths often imply that a special bond is formed between woman and child. On his famous homecoming after a decade-long absence, the first person to recognise Odysseus was his former wet nurse, Eurycleia. I think of Kahlo's painting, the absence of palpable emotion and the unsettling feelings this provokes; the paradox between oxytocin flowing from the nipples and the blankness of both faces. I think back to Hera and Juno, the divine wives whose milk was taken from them as they slept. We know that Hercules obtains immortality, that the galaxy is created and lilies flower, but what happened to Juno? To Hera? What happens afterwards?

Bengali writer and activist Mahasweta Devi considered the aftermath after a lifetime of breastfeeding. The English title of her short story, 'Breast-Giver', emphasises the centrality of the female body and avoids the euphemistic term 'wet nurse'. Devi's protagonist, Jashoda, was a wet nurse for thirty years, during which time she fed a total of fifty babies: twenty of her own (Jashoda can't recall when her husband didn't 'drill her body like a geologist in a darkness lit only by an oil lamp') and thirty more belonging to the rich family for whom she worked. The name Jashoda references Yashoda, the foster-mother of Krishna. A twelfth-century South Indian bronze shows Yashoda holding the baby on her lap, hands cupping his head and knees while the child, nursing from one breast, tweaks Yashoda's other nipple, a gesture that will be familiar to breastfeeding mothers. In 'Breast-Giver' Jashoda is described as 'a professional mother', a role that gets folded into broader Indian iconographies of sacred cows and of Mother India. Jashoda's husband gives up work after being gravely injured when the son of the local patriarch runs him over, and Jashoda becomes the breadwinner as wet nurse to the patriarch's ever-expanding family. The family becomes devoted to her, but Jashoda is trapped within the oppressive forces of capitalism and patriarchy. In her introduction critic and translator of the text, Gayatri Chakravorty Spivak, notes that the breast is not symbolic; it is 'a survival object transformed into a commodity'.[10] Spivak also notes the attention this short story brings to wet-nursing as a professional activity, positioned as a commodity. At the end of the story, we find Jashoda after retirement, alone and abandoned by her husband and the extended family she nursed for so many years. She is dying of breast cancer.

In other parts of the world, even prior to the transatlantic slave trade, white travellers to West Africa tended to use animalistic terms to describe the people they encountered, which was a factor in the eventual mass exploitation of Black people, through manual labour and reproduction.[11] Once enslaved in the Americas, lactating African women were often compelled to nurse white babies. One diary entry by a white visitor to the South from 1773 reads, 'I find it common here for people of Fortune to have their young

Children suckled [by enslaved Black women].'[12] Slave masters were heavily involved in making decisions regarding the care of the babies, and would force Black mothers to nurse their children on a schedule that would allow them to also continue manual labour. Wet-nursing was 'a uniquely gendered form of exploitation of the highest order that compromised their motherhood'.[13] And the children of enslaved women were also denied the chance to suckle from their own mothers.

In Toni Morrison's novel *Beloved,* milk becomes a metonym for all the freedoms denied to enslaved people. The plot is driven by the protagonist Sethe's promise that her own children will never be denied that milk. Race and class once again intertwine. Historian Marcus Wood has aptly described the process of enslaved wet-nursing as 'theft', and its multifaceted traumas are forcefully interrogated in *Beloved.* Breastfeeding and the control – or lack thereof – that enslaved women had over their own lactation is used to express the almost unspeakable brutality of enslavement. As Sethe recalls, 'there was no nursing milk to call my own. I know what it is to be without the milk that belongs to you; to have to fight and holler for it, and to have so little left.' Sethe had only been allowed to nurse from her mother for a few weeks. She was then fed by a nursemaid, but only after the slave-owner's children had been nursed first. No longer able to recognise her own mother, Sethe was also unable to satisfy her hunger, either for milk or for an emotional bond.

An act of unimaginable violence centred on the maternal breast propels the narrative. Sethe overhears the white schoolteacher – the sadistic new owner of the plantation – giving a lesson on her, Sethe's, animal characteristics. Later, as she and her family plan to escape the plantation, Sethe is cornered in a barn and viciously assaulted by the schoolteacher's nephews, who pin her down and suckle her milk. Milk her body was making for her child, who she had sent on to freedom ahead of her, and milk for the baby still in her womb. The terrorising force of the assault serves to remind us that there is no part of her body or her being that is sacred to either herself or her children. This violation, witnessed by her husband, causes him to flee into madness and an unknown fate. Sethe escapes with her children, but when the schoolteacher catches up with them and tries to kidnap them back to the plantation, Sethe murders her baby. Horrific as this is, here it is framed as an act of motherly protection, Sethe's only possible course of action to save the child from a lifetime of heinous violence and dehumanisation. Later, when Sethe tries to recount her story to a Black man who also escaped the schoolteacher, we find the impossibility of mutual understanding in the horrors they experienced. He focuses on the physical beatings Sethe endured while pregnant, while she repeats with growing insistence 'and they took my milk!'.

Part 6

BEYOND BABY

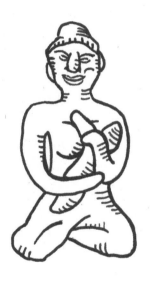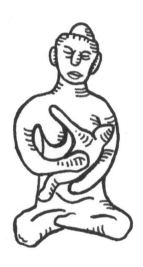

CHAPTER 15

Milk and Charity

A mother touches her fingertips to her face, pulling the skin gently in quiet anguish, a gesture echoed in the furrows across her brow and the frayed hem that frames her elbow. A baby sleeps in her lap. She herself is framed by two children, who bury their heads into her shoulders, the neat, straight edges of their haircuts jarring with the holes in their outsized clothes and grimy skin. You will know this woman's face; the photograph was taken for the United States government and, being copyright-free, it has become one of the most reproduced faces on Earth. The woman is the 'Migrant Mother' and her image crystalised the poverty and desperation of displaced Dust Bowl migrants in the Great Depression. The photograph, taken by Dorothea Lange, first appeared in the *San Francisco News* in March 1936. But it took until 1978 for the world to learn the woman's name: Florence Owens Thompson. She was not in fact a Dust Bowl migrant, but a part-Cherokee widow who had lived in California for roughly a decade, picking vegetables and cotton. When Lange, who was working as a federal photographer, found the family, they were camping with pea-pickers in a frozen field while they waited for their car to be fixed.

Lange made seven photographs of Florence Owens

Thompson and they unfold over a period of time, measured in acts of mothering and increased intimacy. A photograph taken of the family's camp at a distance, three older children posing for the camera. A close-up of Thompson with the baby asleep in her arms. Then, finally, the baby is awake and feeding, Thompson's arms crossed over her body, squashing her daughter to her breast. The worry lines on her face soften. Years later, that baby daughter, Norma, remembered her mother as 'a woman who loved to enjoy life, who loved her children. [. . .] She loved music and she loved to dance. When I look at that photo of Mother, it saddens me. That's not how I like to remember her.'[1] But the world will now always recall Thompson as the worried mother, staving off destitution.

Breastfeeding in this context of poverty and displacement stands for fortitude, the image-makers assured of the cultural universality of the mother and child, certain their audience would understand an image of breastfeeding as an act of maternal love and sacrifice, underscoring the dire circumstances families found themselves in. As Marta Zarzycka notes in her exploration of gender and war imagery, it is photographs of mothers with children that communicate the precarity of the plight of refugees and displaced peoples.[2] In 1980, David Burnett won the World Press Photo Contest with an image taken a year previously of a Cambodian woman waiting at a food distribution centre for refugees fleeing the Khmer Rouge. Emerging from the blackness of the woman's clothing are two very tiny bare feet. Once you notice them, the image takes on a new charge; the jolt of very new, fresh life creates a greater urgency. In April 1999, *Time* magazine covered the plight of Kosovo Albanians who were walking into Macedonia to escape war. The cover was a close-up photograph of a young mother in a thick coat, walking towards the camera holding a baby concealed in blankets to her bare breast. The white of her headscarf reflects the whites of her knuckles as she grips her baby's fleece blanket fiercely. There is snow on the ground, and behind her, slightly out of focus, a long line of refugees demonstrates the scale of the crisis, distilled into this image of maternal suffering.

The Migrant Mother became the symbol of what John Steinbeck called the Harvest Gypsies in his essays for the *San Francisco News*. When the essays were gathered into a collection called *Their Blood is Strong* in 1938, the cover image was another photograph of a breastfeeding mother taken by Lange. A young mother is perched on a camp bed, an almost-naked infant nursing on her lap. The child tugs at the nipple with their mouth and pushes into the breast with a fist. Mother and child both look into the camera. She holds a protective arm across the child's body, the right angle of her elbow perfectly mirroring the child's. A pair of bare feet hang off the bed in the right-hand corner of the image; we assume they belong to a man, exhausted and hopeless.

I now know my desire to continue breastfeeding did not spring from nowhere and that my unconscious was operating at a cultural level, drawing on all the symbolism and allegory that feeds into our ideas of female bodies and mothers and life and death. It came from the art I'd seen and the books I'd read. And perhaps there was also an instinctual drive, precipitated by hormones, to sustain life. Milk extinguishes the flames of death again and again. This is one of the reasons that the metaphorical and symbolic potential of breastfeeding is abundant. The *Madonna lactans*, with her swollen breasts, has been read as exemplary of the selflessness, love and nurturing of mothering, neutralising the profound power of the maternal into symbols of divine love and salvation. In the twelfth and thirteenth centuries, breast milk was a vital metaphor for the Christian church. When Saint Catherine of Alexandria was executed, milk, not blood, spurted from her severed neck (The same was said to have happened to Saint Paul the Apostle when he was executed for his beliefs). This is exemplified in the writing of seventeenth-century English religious leaders, who compared eternal bliss to the happy baby at his mother's breast, weaning to the helplessness of spiritual loss. In Puritan New England, male preachers employed maternal imagery, describing themselves as 'the breasts of God', whose Word was like milk, passing through and out of the preacher's body for the nourishment of his faithful.[3]

Centuries later, Florence Owens Thompson was aware of the cultural milieu in which her image found itself, in particular the maternal and religious imagery later used by Steinbeck in his novels; she said, 'When Steinbeck wrote *The Grapes of Wrath* about those people living under the bridge at Bakersfield – at one time we lived under that bridge. It was the same story. Didn't even have a tent then, just a ratty old quilt.'[4] The novel was published in 1939 and follows the Joad family as they travel from Oklahoma to California in search of work after their farm is repossessed by the bank. As the extended family migrate west along Route 66, Rose of Sharon's husband abandons them. California is saturated with workers, who are cruelly exploited, and the family exists on the edge of starvation. Throughout the book Rose, who is pregnant, remains steadfastly focused on a future far removed from the destitution the family presently finds themselves in, a future where 'the baby'll have all new stuff [. . .] we want it nice for the baby'. She smiles often.

Sadly, life and death conspire differently and Rose's baby is stillborn. The final scene in the book sees the family taking shelter from winter rains in an old barn, alongside a young

boy and his father, who is so malnourished he is on the
brink of death. The book ends with Rose of Sharon breastfeeding the man alone, in a barn surrounded by flooded
cotton fields. We are given brief details of the intimacy of
that act; that she supports his head with her hand, combs
her fingers gently through his hair as one might nurse a
child, and, finally, that her 'lips came together and smiled
mysteriously'.

Steinbeck drew on potent imagery for the denouement
of his Great Depression novel. In the European context,
we can trace this imagery back to the first century AD,
when the Roman historian Valerius Maximus included two
transgressive acts of nursing in his *Factorum et dictorum
memorabilium libri*, or *Memorable Doings and Sayings*.
His works were among the most copied Latin prose texts in
the medieval period, indicating their popularity and influence throughout the centuries. In a chapter called 'Of Piety
towards Parents', several examples are given of a woman
breastfeeding a parent who has found themselves in un-
fortunate circumstance. In the first example, an unnamed
woman is condemned to death but her jailer takes pity on
her and saves her from execution. He allows her daughter
to visit, each time ensuring she isn't bringing food to her
mother. What the jailer neglects, however, is the nourishing
potential of the daughter's body; she surreptitiously nurses
her mother. On discovering the deceit, the authorities are
so struck by such a 'novel and remarkable spectacle', they
pardon the old woman and release her from jail. In the
second account, a young woman named Pero feeds her
father Cimon, who also languishes on the brink of starvation in a prison. Valerius writes that 'Pero took his head to
her breast and nursed him, as if he were a baby.'[5]

This motif has for centuries been interpreted as a tale
of filial piety; it became known as Roman Charity and, by

the Renaissance, these stories had become infused with a religious tone. Just as the pagan Isis prefigured Mary, so Pero came to embody the specifically Christian virtue of Charity. The devotion of Pero to her father was expanded into the image of Mary, the mother who offered the faithful nourishment, symbolised by her breast milk. The earliest-known of the countless depictions of this story comes from a fresco from Pompeii, in which a seated woman looks down towards the emaciated male who feeds from her breast. Caravaggio included the scene in his 1607 painting *The Seven Works of Mercy*. Putting his famous chiaroscuro to perfect use, Caravaggio illuminates each of the human examples of merciful acts, as the rest of the composition broods in darkness. Pero and her father, representing the virtue of visiting the imprisoned and feeding the hungry, dominate the right third of the pictorial field. She hurriedly leans into the prison window as her father stretches his head through the bars to feed. She looks over her shoulder, alert to the action behind her and, perhaps, fearing she may be caught in this transgressive act of salvation. Drops of milk catch in her father's grey beard. Rubens painted four versions of Roman Charity, the first of which he created in 1612, adhering to the conventions of this concept with a young woman kneeling on a squalid straw floor, guiding her nipple into the mouth of a lethargic yet muscular man who slumps against her breast. His solid biceps and rippling torso do not suggest a man much starved. Less interested in portraying the *Madonna lactans*, Rubens instead focuses on the act of nursing as symbolic of Christian charity, 'recasting the everyday activity of feeding as a redemptive good work'.[6] In *Cimon and Pero* (c.1625) a seated woman in red looks away as her father, hands shackled behind his back, leans into her breast. Her eyes may be averted, but her hand rests gently on his naked back, her other hand shaping her breast to his mouth. Two guards secretly observe the scene through the bars of the window.

My first encounter with an image of breastfeeding as filial piety took place one cloudy afternoon in Singapore. I was in the city for a conference and decided to spend a free afternoon wandering through Haw Par Villa, a cultural village built in 1937 by Aw Boon Haw, dubbed the Tiger Balm King after making millions from developing the herbal ointment. The site is a sprawling, eclectic mix of dioramas and life-sized statues, and is perhaps best known for its 'Ten Courts of Hell', a 60-metre trail that leads the visitor through a tunnel where we are surrounded by stagings of violent and horribly specific punishments for crimes. But I remember being most taken by a life-sized diorama of a woman breastfeeding an elderly grandmother, her pink dress open as she cups her breast for the white-haired woman who kneels before her. A baby lies fussing on the floor and a small child plays with a ball. I returned to my hotel later that evening and read about the *Twenty-Four Filial Exemplars*, written during the Yuan dynasty (1260–1368). One of the examples tells the story of Madam Zhangsun, an old woman who has lost her teeth. Unable to eat, her daughter-in-law breastfeeds her for years. Before her death, Madam Zhangsun tells her family she can never repay her daughter-in-law's devotion and, therefore, the family should treat her kindly.

My own curiosity but also uneasiness about this imagery points to the general cultural confusion that lactation presents. Take Barbara Krafft's 1797 version of filial piety, in which any pretence at cleaving to the original Pero story is abandoned. Krafft, best known for her portrait of Wolfgang Amadeus Mozart, has recently found new fame as an internet meme; her depiction of Roman Charity has gone viral thanks to its jarring composition and ambiguous sexual undertones. The father is no longer languishing in a squalid prison cell but instead sits back against plump green cushions on a gilded chair. He is frail, his milky-pale skin the fashionable colour for the wealthy of the period. Beside him on the occasional table sits a teacup and a half-emptied crystal bottle of alcohol or perhaps medicine. A younger woman, who we assume is his daughter, is similarly pale but with a slight flush of pink. She stands behind the arm of the chair, holding her bare breast towards the man's face. The setting is startling, but the composition also dovetails with other versions of Pero and Cimon in that both look directly towards the viewer. A slight smile plays across the father's face; he is unabashed. The young woman looks uncertain. With this direct gaze we, the viewer, are invited into a scene that is neither desperate nor holy. Beyond the gesture of leaning towards the father, there is no suggestion of breastfeeding, no droplet of milk that would indicate this is a scene of lactation. The transgressive nature of the image is, perhaps, tempered when we learn the figures in the image are not father and daughter, but husband and wife, Count Franz de Paula Graf von Hartig and his wife Eleanore. The bare breast is now erotically charged without complication, and we are instead presented with what might be a scene of consensual adults partaking in lactation play, itself an often unspoken fetish. It's easy to see why this image could take on multiple lives online, provoking shock, intrigue and disgust in equal measure.

Lactation can be a metaphor for godliness and a practice of piety, while at the same time being viewed as gross and provoking squeamishness. No wonder the topic of milk spills out across feminist discourses, vexing the terms of engagement and leaving us all in a highly confused – and confusing – cultural bind, where the physiological and socially constructed meet in an emotional, corporeal milieu.

Or, to quote Linda Blum, 'breastfeeding provides a wonderful lens magnifying the cracks and fractures in our construction of the [. . .] mother. As an experience of intense interdependence between mother and infant, breastfeeding is easily romanticised; yet, at the same time, the present social context makes breastfeeding extremely difficult for women'.[7]

Legendary tales of interfamilial nursing instil a sense of discomforting taboo. Yet these are cultural sidenotes. The dominant cultural dichotomy between the sexual and maternal breast is more enfeebling, preventing us from thinking critically about the intersections of gender, sexuality, maternity and parenthood. Today, confusion around breastfeeding bodies proliferates; we are told that it is 'best for baby', yet breasts are hyper-sexualised and bodily fluids are taboo. Where does that leave the person who inhabits a body that functions and desires across these binaries?

CHAPTER 16

Community

The thread of motherhood came to me early, when I was not even two months pregnant. These are the silent, secretive weeks of nascent parenthood. We had only told close family because I was afraid that if I spoke of the baby – conjured him into existence with words – he would disappear. His heart had only just begun to beat and my body vibrated to all these invisible unknowns. My body was taking me places that my partner couldn't follow or understand, however hard he tried. All he could do was bring me offerings of bland carbohydrates and watch as I retreated far into myself by myself; yet for the first time, I was not ever alone.

In the West in recent centuries, pregnancy has been characterised as a time of passive waiting until 'her time comes'. But that veil of quiet expectation conceals eruptions within. Beneath my skin, the skeins of biology, hormones and culture were stirring a raw, primal urge inside me. These were also unspeakable, but their vibrations called out to the women who had come before me. The need to be with them was so strong that I fantasised about moving next door to my mum; on family visits I shuffled to sit closer to my aunt; I called my sister daily. My beloved grandmother, who had passed away eight years previously, was more frequently in my thoughts too, and I could feel the softness of her hands on my arm, the smooth skin of her cheek brushing against mine. Despite the vast differences in the contexts of our pregnancies, I knew there would be enough continuity for her to guide me through this passage. I felt a fresh tug in my heart, the pull of a new thread that connected me to her, that hadn't existed before, until eventually I sensed that I was being stitched into a network that spanned the whole of human time. Perhaps it is no wonder I feel the pull of Louise Bourgeois with her textiles and spiders, of Indonesian bronzes of women at a loom. As I lay alone at night, I heard these women call back to me.

Their call stayed with me as my body morphed and the baby became real. Periodically, the eruptions happening within found a way out, manifesting in early-pregnancy anxiety complete with vividly intrusive and disturbing thoughts. I was swiftly appointed a midwife from the perinatal mental health team and she would come to my flat, taking blood samples as I sat on my sofa, my rescue cat nuzzling my side. Soon, those ugly thoughts dissipated, as my belly grew bigger and the love and hope that had always resided with me felt safe enough to emerge. I welcomed my routine hospital appointments, but only when they were with women: I bristled when male consultants dismissed my questions, feeling myself grow smaller as they talked over me, their eyes barely lifting from the notes on their desk to meet mine. Sure, they were well-trained. And absolutely, neither a uterus nor a baby makes a woman. In Maggie Nelson's definition of womanhood, it is a communality of living – and sometimes creating life – within a patriarchy. The *simpatico* I felt among women was not ignited by body parts, but by a deeply shared sense of community, of not-maleness.

Communality. Women sitting beside women. In Si Satchanalai, Thailand, there is a cache of glazed ceramic figurines depicting breastfeeding women. The small figures, modelled by hand, measure around 11cm tall and date from between 1350 and 1550 CE. Their attire indicates that they are intended to represent mortal women rather than divinities. I find an image of a pair of these green-glazed figures in the online archive of San Francisco's Asian Art Museum. Artefacts such as these are usually photographed individually, stark within the blank background of the photograph. But these two have been placed side by side, and I wonder if whoever posed them recognised the potential loneliness of parenting and the power of being in a space with another person engaged in the same activity as you. Each woman holds her baby to her left breast, the right hand supporting the baby's bottom. Mirroring this gesture, each baby's left arm reaches up as if trying to embrace their mother. The women are seated, one with crossed legs, the other with knees bent and legs tucked to her right side, both traditional ways of sitting to ensure one does not show the soles of one's feet – a taboo in Southeast Asia. One woman smiles broadly, but her companion looks more unsure, tentative. I like to imagine the woman smiling is a seasoned parent, seated with a first-time mother.

Similar figures, some of which are now headless, have been found across Asia, from Java to the Philippines and Japan, where they appear to have had some ritual function, perhaps as burial objects. Based on archaeological finds, some scholars speculate that a ritual decapitation of these maternal figures was carried out to ensure safe childbirth. However, there is no textual evidence to support such activity and it is just as likely that the weight of the mother's head made it liable to break from the delicate ceramic neck. But despite their ubiquity, there is little written on this. As I pore over research relating to ceramics of this period, I find that meticulous attention has been paid to male and mythical figurines but there is scant consideration of the women. Perhaps, because mothering has been assumed to be only biophysical, simply a 'natural' part of a woman's life, these statues have attracted little curiosity, especially when overshadowed by great men and kings. Yet, these figures give us tantalising glimpses of the daily life of mothers; one breastfeeding figurine has a bulging cheek, indicating she is chewing betel nut. Another woman wrestles with two infants clamouring at her chest.

We will never know who sculpted these images or their precise reasons for doing so, but, in the end, the fact of their manufacture indicates that these were important things to capture in material form. Was making these figures a ritual in itself? I like to imagine that they were made by women, that their fingers modelled the clay just as women in the Indus Valley may have pressed their fingers into breasts and babies a millennia before, just as Ashlee Wells Jackson revealed maternal bodies and babies in a darkroom centuries later, just as Catherine Opie fashioned her self-portrait.

Representation can build communities; it can be a gift that says *I see you*. Imagine yourself as a new mother, navigating your new identities and roles, taking a small figurine of a woman who looks like you – chewing betel, breastfeeding a baby – and placing it somewhere in your home. It makes you feel your efforts are recognised each time you glance at it. It makes you feel valued. It allows you to look back at yourself and embody all the mothers that came before. But, in our world where caregivers are under-rewarded and breastfeeding comes swathed in taboos, I wonder how lactating women are supposed to work out how to represent themselves, especially publicly? For many women today, community and representation are found in private online support groups, social media and local community centres. Such spaces suffer from chronic underinvestment, but they are crucial places for women to tell their stories, as well as allowing space for communal support and the sharing of wisdom passed from parent to parent. These spaces are vital repositories of feminine knowledge.

This knowledge, shared, constitutes a kind of 'folk' knowledge. As a lecturer, I spend hours discussing with students how the European Enlightenment and imperialism conspired to set up certain kinds of knowledge as superior. In Europe, and later across the globalised world, other kinds of knowledge have been lost through the medicalisation of birth and early infancy. That's not to say modern medicine is bad or wrong; I am beyond grateful that I gave birth to my baby in the time and place that I did. But outside of these structures, there are certain kinds of wisdom that women pass to their daughters and around and within their communities.

To understand the benefits of communal knowledge, we can look at what happens when it disappears. For example, in the modern world the loss of community and intergenerational ties that occurs with urbanisation can negatively impact successful breastfeeding. Nomajoni Ntombela, chair of the African office of the International Baby Food Action Network, cites the loss of social networks as a factor in the decrease in breastfeeding rates across Africa. Breastfeeding is not necessarily intuitive, but for many it is a learned skill requiring the kind of knowledge that is passed from generation to generation. Within Europe, the decline in breastfeeding in the twentieth century means that, even though rates are improving now, there has been a loss of knowledge and understanding, a narrowing of what is deemed acceptable and proper.[1]

In addition to knowledge specifically about how breastfeeding works and the practicalities of getting it right, other forms of knowledge are passed on to women throughout their perinatal period. As well as offering practical support, small rituals or whispered words of wisdom can help bind the new parent into a stronger community network. For example, in the early 1970s Marie Walter enlisted the help of La Leche League to speak to nursing mothers and record breastfeeding beliefs that were preserved in oral traditions. She corresponded with mothers across the USA and five other countries and recorded tales of the kinds of food women should consume, along with stories of sympathetic magic.[2] In eastern Kentucky it was reported that if the mother witnesses a death she should not nurse soon after because the baby will die immediately. A mother in Brazil recounts that if a mother steps on breast milk that has spilled on the floor, her supply will dry up instantly. In Sri Lanka, the placenta is hung on a fig tree; this is believed to stimulate the mother's milk production. This information is as much about building bonds and forming continuities as it is about anything else. I was told that fennel helped increase milk supply, and happily drank endless cups of tea made from the stuff. The same recommendation is found in a medieval manuscript that dates from at least the twelfth century, along with advice to consume lettuce, cumin, ginger and white pepper. Of course, I attribute my increase in milk supply to modern breast pumps, nationalised healthcare and relatively recent research on breast-milk production. At the same time, the durability of fennel's reputation in this area demonstrates that many women have worried about milk supply, at many different times and in many different places. As another herbal teabag stews in the mug beside me, I reflect again on those who came before me, with their similar worries and fears to mine. Their similar small rituals, their talismans of hope. The things that we cling to for encouragement.

For much of history, birthing and post-partum women

would have been attended to by a network of female family members. In patrilineal families this would often be the mother-in-law and sisters-in-law, neighbours and midwives, the latter of whom were usually married or widowed women whose children were older and who were thus both experienced and freer from domestic caring duties of their own. It was a period of 'female solidarity'. The only exception to this would be royal births, when ensuring the legitimacy of a potential heir meant the presence of the king and high court officials to ensure the correct baby had come from the correct uterus.[3]

Some of this wisdom remains, finding a way through and between, like buddleia growing between concrete blocks. In the UK, nursing mothers will be told to put cabbage leaves in their bra to ease engorgement, or to dry out milk when a mother no longer wants or needs to breastfeed, a treatment also known in China. In southern India and Malaysia, engorgement is helped by spreading jasmine flowers over the breast and holding them in place with loose cloth. Who collects these small, white flowers? I picture an aunt or a husband leaving home at dusk, just as the jasmine buds open and release their intoxicating aroma: floral, yet animalic. This duality seems fitting: sensual and intimate, yet warm and fragile. I feel short-changed for having had to cup my breasts in thick, sulphurous cabbage leaves when I could have been enveloped in blossoms.

But none of this is mere window dressing. These things have been rigorously tried and tested and peer reviewed; studies concur that jasmine flowers and cabbage leaves are an effective cure for engorgement or for drying up milk. Yet putting scientific assurances aside, our collective mothers knew what to share with us, what knowledge to preserve. When a husband was instructed to go out to buy cabbage or jasmine flowers, this was not an idle trip. There was a purpose to it, a gesture of tenderness – and, perhaps, a way to get them out of the house.

Why would I doubt that our ancestors knew where to look within their own backyards for the relief of elemental ailments? Why was I surprised when my Norwegian friend told me that women there still sometimes use limpet shells to soothe their chapped nipples? Patella vulgata are found along shorelines from the Arctic Circle down to the coast of Great Britain, and as far south as Portugal. Scandinavian women have known about these for centuries at least, and they are still recommended for nursing mothers, who are advised to wear them between feeds to catch leaks and protect nipples from rubbing against fabric. Maybe Botticelli was on to something with his *Birth of Venus*. These shells make me think of the cleansing salt air and the breath of Zephyr gently helping Venus float towards the shore, as she emerges from the ocean in a scallop shell into the warming embrace of the thick cloak held by another of the Hora, representing spring and renewal. The curve of a cabbage leaf that hugs the hard breast tissue; a heady carpet of luxurious jasmine blossom; the perfectly shaped pyramid of a limpet shell cupping a cracked nipple, catching leaking breast milk that will heal the nipple. And all of these make sense. And together, they all suggest a woman held by a community.

My passage into parenthood was marked by encounters where I felt a thread of connection back to women in the past. One such time was an early-September evening, shortly after my son had been discharged from hospital with slow weight gain. We had been told by the hospital lactation consultant to see someone privately if possible. The idea of having a specialist come into our space with the time to really sit with us was highly appealing. We checked our bank balance and I scoured recommendations and reviews online, then made the phone call. Within twenty-four hours she appeared, ushering in a degree of relief simply with her presence. She was confident and authoritative, as if knowing that women so close to the end of their tether need a firm hold.

She sat on the sofa and took a brief history. My story tumbled out, as fragmented as you read it here. She spent fifteen minutes carefully examining my son, although within seconds of probing his tiny mouth with a gloved finger she confidently detected tongue-tie. The membrane on the floor of his tongue was too tight, restricting his tongue's movement, which resulted in a shallow and less effective latch. She could cut it for us right there. I snapped on the reading lamp and my partner laid a red blanket on the sofa as we made long, searching eye contact with each other, trying to read the other's mind to decide if we were doing the right thing here, with this woman we found on the internet. When she left the room to wash her hands, we whispered to one another: are we crazy to let this woman cut our son? Should we just have faith? I was too tired and too desperate to do otherwise. I was out of options. She returned and laid out surgical gloves and a sterile pack of scissors. It won't hurt him, she reassured us. The air was thick – and why do I remember mist? It felt like a ritual, emotions heightened by exhaustion, desperation and vulnerability. The only crying in the room came from my usually stoic partner; he said he saw the membrane snap like a tree branch.

But the tension was cut too and there was calm. My son was quiet and ready to feed. She carried the baby to me, and he latched deeply and easily as she gave gentle pointers on position and how to shape my breast. But what I remember most is a reverential peace. I felt for that moment like the Holy Mother, finally. She spent a total of two hours with us, at a cost of £200.

Ancient medical sources refer to cutting this membrane

under the tongue if it is too thick and restrictive. In the Middle Ages, midwives would snip the membrane with a sharp fingernail. Nowadays, there is conflicting information and advice as to whether tongue-tie affects feeding. Does this signify a loss of knowledge in a more medicalised world? Or is it an unnecessary intervention? How am I to know? Does transmission of such wisdom represent an initiation of sorts: you are now a mother and belong to a new subset of the community? How are these bonds forged? How have our communities shifted from local kinship bonds to the amorphous space of social media? What has been lost? And what has been gained?

When I was five months pregnant my sister and I flew to Marrakech. This was my third time in the city, and I knew it would provide the comfort of the familiar along with the distraction of the unfamiliar. We spent long afternoons sitting on sunny rooftops drinking mint tea and nibbling olives. She was my mirror, able to express palpable excitement over the baby, the kind of excitement I couldn't yet articulate. I luxuriated in the joy and optimism she radiated. An introvert, I found comfort in retreating inwards, sensing the larger community that I carried within myself. While pregnant I could lie in silence in a yoga room filled with other pregnant people, our breathing slowing as we each tuned in to our babies and our bodies. Support could be abstract. But later on, once my baby was born, I needed tangible community support. I was a breastfeeding neophyte and this made me ashamed. Ashamed because, no matter how many people showed me how to hold him or told me how good my latch was, it still wasn't working. It felt like each person had one small piece of a puzzle but no one knew what the whole picture should look like, so I was just bashing pieces together to try to make them fit.

Yet I was still compelled to be with other parents. Whenever I could, I'd push the pram to local breastfeeding cafés in community centres or the public library. At some, volunteers would bring us hot, sweet tea in travel mugs as we tried to get comfy in plastic chairs. They would ask us how we were doing and offer words of encouragement. I assumed that they were all so pro-breastfeeding because they'd had nothing but wonderful experiences, but in fact most volunteers I spoke to had gone through many difficulties themselves. I'd chat with new mums, safe in the knowledge that we were all there seeking help. And then I would trudge home, closing the door behind me. The atomised mother, the locked-down parent, sitting enveloped in the worry that only swells up in the middle of the night. (Writing this book feels a bit like new motherhood: when I planned the research, I was expecting to visit archives, galleries, to handle objects, look at painterly brushstrokes, sip coffee with women whose experiences mirrored and diverged from mine. Instead, like everyone in Britain, I am at home, living life through a screen, casting about for something to grasp – a footnote in a book, an etching that has been digitised – something to distract me from the physical isolation.)

Aside from the ceramic figures, I am struck by how few paintings I encounter of women breastfeeding communally. But I do find flashes of the kind of support required to maintain breastfeeding. *Good Neighbours*, an oil on panel from the late eighteenth century by Dutch painter Johannes Christiaan Janson, depicts a young woman seated next to an unmade box bed breastfeeding a rosy-cheeked baby, with a small boy sitting at her feet reading a book. A woman, likely a maid, stands beside her offering her a drink and I recall the desperate, relentless thirst. If you take one thing from this book, let it be this: whenever you see someone breastfeeding or expressing milk, bring them a cool glass of water.

*

I had been told to expect loneliness during the night feeds, and broadly this was true. The enormous weight of responsibility somehow felt heavier, the uncertainties in my head more numerous. Sitting in bed, I would think of all the other parents waking in the dead of night to attend to a mewling newborn. I shared in their exhaustion, their love, perhaps the swollen sensation in their breasts, the damp patch on their nightdress. All this time and all this energy to sustain life.

But when the door shuts and the curtains close, another space can open with the swipe of a finger. Via the phone in my hand, I had access to the largest community of women in history, sharing stories on blogs or advice on forums. The internet allows for support networks that reach beyond one's own neighbourhood or community, with the potential for hundreds of women to answer your cries for help at 3 a.m. This happened to me. I returned from that hospital with a breast pump and a tub of formula, and retreated with my baby to a crumpled bed. The regime made it near-impossible to leave the house and I was reclusive and afraid. 'Will I ever breastfeed my son again?' I posed to a Mumsnet forum, complete with a long, desperate account of our troubles. I braced myself for condemnation or judgement. Either for failing to breastfeed properly, or for turning my nose up at formula. Instead, I was overwhelmed by the chorus of women who took the time to reply. Each shared their experiences, passed on recommendations for further support, or simply told me I was doing an excellent job. Recalling these words from strangers still moves me to tears. It wasn't just their advice and support, but the experience of feeling seen and held, even in the anonymous digital sphere.

This was to be my one and only foray into posting on Mumsnet. But for other women, the internet offers longer-term solace and companionship. I spoke to one woman who had relocated due to her husband's job. Without physical access to her usual friendship groups, she joined a forum thread for expectant parents due in the same month. They shared pregnancy updates, sought recommendations for cots and eventually swapped birth stories. It was the kind of place where someone could describe their episiotomy stitches and no one would flinch. From the forum, they moved to a Facebook group that, eight years on, has a core of around fifty mothers from a wide range of cultures, now scattered across the globe and still supporting one another with the project of raising children. This same woman had joined a fantastic peer support breastfeeding group in southeast London when she had her first baby. They met weekly. Although the polystyrene cups of tea and camaraderie were appreciated, she described just sitting with other mums as the most amazing aspect of the group. Being together in a space. This had the added benefit of allowing women to share their positive breastfeeding stories in all their variety. How individual babies prefer to position themselves, different durations of feeds, how each of us is unique.

But once those real-life groups scattered, as they eventually and inevitably do when people return to work or leave the area, online spaces provided the same visibility of breastfeeding. In her parenting forum, this woman felt, there was far less judgement, the relative anonymity and geographical and temporal distance between members resulting in less apparent insecurity in sharing intimate details of family life. Being able to take the time to think and craft thoughtful responses to people's posts or questions also made the space more helpful and supportive.

In the absence of breastfeeding in the wider cultural landscape, these spaces are sacred. Other online groups are by turns intimate, supportive and playful. I'm still a member of

a group dedicated to sharing breastfeeding-friendly clothing, and my feed is full of women nursing with confidence
and looking fantastic. They share advice on how to tailor
a wedding dress so babies can feed, or answer heartbreak-
ing questions such as: 'What can I wear to a funeral so I
can still feed my three-week-old?' Researcher Aleksandra
Maria Męcińska describes these online and offline spaces
and groups as the 'lactosphere', a space that is

> both local and global, made up of organisations and
> individuals all advocating for breastfeeding. The con-
> nections between them are ones of cooperation and
> proximity, affinity and connection, mutual awareness,
> or recirculation ('sharing') of objects [. . .] It consists
> of real-life entities and their online avatars – websites,
> blogs, profiles, screen names ('nicks').[4]

The ability to give language to experience is also heightened
in these spaces. Zainab Yate, author of *When Breastfeeding Sucks*, describes the 'private-speak' and 'public-speak'
of women who experience breastfeeding aversion. Within
the safe spaces of the aversion community, women describe
their experiences in visceral and raw terms. They know they
are among people who will understand and can express
'a myriad of emotions that those outside the group who
don't understand experience would find really shocking,
but which others in the group would be able to empathise
and say, Oh, you know, I've been there and you might feel
awful and these are the things that you could try to do'.[5]
But within more public realms, their descriptions tend to be
more diluted and palatable. They temper the raw emotion
to protect themselves and/or the listener.

Support from strangers exists in other places too. Under-
funded places. One afternoon, about ten weeks after my

son was born, I fell apart. That morning we went to a breastfeeding peer support group in a community centre not far from our home. We signed the visitor register at reception, walked past the community food bank, and into a large room of plastic chairs and nervous parents, where we were welcomed with a broad smile and ushered to a seat. A sports bottle of water appeared on the table in front of me. Weights were lifted. A helpful volunteer sat beside me and showed me how to better position the baby. It worked and I was elated. He latched deeply and my own pain faded. At 10 a.m. we had to vacate the space. I had been awake for hours already and the rest of the day loomed before me. By the time we settled down for the long afternoon feed, everything had gone wrong again; it hurt and the baby was fussy. Sitting in the depression at the end of the sofa formed by many hours of nursing and napping, I sobbed. And I called the breastfeeding helpline. The woman who answered listened patiently as I explained our predicament and the hopelessness of it all. Then, calmly, she talked me through the positioning of the baby and I finally – finally – managed to explain that I just didn't understand the nose-to-nipple instruction. In the background I could hear the sound of young children and the whirr of her washing machine. She talked me through my anatomy, my baby's anatomy, with me staring down at my nipples in confusion. And then, it clicked. He latched and fed. She told me I was doing a wonderful job. She told me to take it one feed at a time. She said goodbye and I never even found out her name.

Communities can be the armour we wear.

I can forget this when I think too much about perceived judgement from other mothers, mothers who made different choices in different circumstances. We are told to forget this when we are encouraged to compare ourselves to images of others on social media, all nuance flattened out. We are easier to sell to if we are fragmented, from ourselves and each other. If we feel pitched against one another then we can find ourselves wanting, and if we are wanting we can become insecure, and if we are insecure we are less powerful and more susceptible. I return to the stories told by friends of what made them feel comfortable as new breastfeeding mothers, and again and again it was the presence of other women, sometimes other breastfeeding mothers, but often simply other women, especially older women who perhaps gave off a maternal vibe. 'If I was surrounded I felt protected.' There is power in our bodies, in our visibility, in our very being. We gather and hold space, even without realising it.

I keep coming back to the idea of threads and weaving, as if trying to construct something bigger out of my own experience. Because milk – in whichever way it is delivered – is the white ink that writes our origin stories, which binds us all together generation after generation, woman with woman, community with community. In 2003 Louise Bourgeois made one of several works entitled *The Good Mother*. It is a title she used for works in many mediums: bronze, gouache on paper, print and collages, all of pregnant bodies, large breasts expelling silvery-white fluids, the edges of multiple breasts bleeding out into the page. The 2003 version takes the form of a pink textile figure kneeling on a steel pedestal. I have spoken about this figure before, but I can't stop coming back to her. She looks like an unfinished stuffed toy with no hair; the stitches across her body look like scars. Five white threads extend from her nipples to five metal bobbins, spaced in a semicircle in front of her, already wound with thick spools of thread. There are multiple ways that I could read this work. The sterility of the pedestal, the inhumanity of the figure tethered to the spools, producing and producing milk, like a cow in an industrial dairy. I think about the women in Cambodia producing breast milk for export to a foreign market, milk spooling out and away, but ultimately to whom and where?

But what also compels me to return to The *Good Mother* is the connection and community I read into her, even though she is alone. In Buddhist contexts, statues of the Buddha are ritually consecrated, to imbue the stone or cement or metal with ephemeral Buddhahood. To do this, monks each hold a sacred thread, which is wrapped round the new statue and an older statue. The thread transfers sacred power from the statues to the monks and vice versa.[6] I doubt Bourgeois was referencing Buddhist consecration ceremonies, but when I look at her work, I see thick white threads that bind us across time. Milk that can build communities, one feed at a time.

Because if milk is about anything it is about community, starting from the community of two – the mother and child – and growing out into networks at microlocal, local, national levels, levels that can transcend beyond borders and even through time. To know our histories is to know ourselves.

EPILOGUE

Ending was easier than starting. We became breastfeeding virtuosos just as we started introducing other foods. My son took to solids with gusto, sucking on moist broccoli, smashing raspberries into his mouth, and painstakingly chasing peas across his high-chair tray. He started drinking cups of cows' milk, unperturbed by and accepting of the differences between this milk and 'mummy milk'. By the time he was one, I felt entirely relieved of providing all his nourishment. Breastfeeding instead became a means to express aspects of our relationship and our moods. There are many threads that connect us to our children and milk was one of ours.

Like a yo-yo, he moved further and further away from me, but we always spooled back together eventually. These moments could be precious. Sometimes my son would lie cradled and outsized in my arms, his flesh utterly relaxed and eyes softly gazing at mine. Other times he'd sit on my lap, legs straddling my hips, arms wrapped tightly round me, head buried in flesh, my nose buried in his hair. This allowed for maximum bodily contact, and I like to imagine it provided a warm, contained space for him when the world he was exploring more and more independently became too overwhelming. This time also gave me glimpses of his life beyond me: the scent of his childminder's body lotion, a smear of felt-tip pen on his elbow, the faint smell of woodchips from the playground, damp saltiness from an afternoon nap. Other times, he would feed standing up, his head turned upside down to latch on, like an acrobat, arms swinging as he multitasked; breastfeeding just one activity of many, my body no longer an extension of his, but an extension of the world-as-playground. Over time he started asking for it less and I tried to stop offering.

Immediately after my son was born, I was bewildered and out of control, and wanted to breastfeed as it was the 'best' thing I could do. Yet it was impossible to maintain the perfectionism that has blighted me for as long as I can remember. It was impossible because my son is an independent entity. Strange then, that mutual feelings of possession are often seen as a 'normal' component of new parenthood. When he was born my early thoughts were 'he's not mine', which terrified me. I was sure a sense of possession was an integral part of maternal love. Then one evening, looking at him asleep beside me, I heard my voice say, 'You are not mine, but you are of me.' And now, months and months later, breastfeeding was still our beautiful thing, even as we were two people with lives diverging imperceptibly. Our wants and needs couldn't always align. There were times I felt touched out, the thought of sharing my body with another too much. Sometimes his demand for milk felt too abrupt – rude even – and if I tried to distract him or refuse, he would claw and tug his way into my shirt. But, as the psychoanalysts knew, there is always a cruelty to weaning. In *Romeo and Juliet*, the nurse recalls in detail Juliet's weaning at age three, suggesting it was a significant and emotionally charged event for them both. The nurse remembers where precisely she was sat, where the parents were (absent), and that she applied wormwood to her nipple, its bitter taste repelling and enraging the infant. I remember my toddler son, so distressed, grabbing at my shirt with force, searching for my breast. Yes, there was a hint of menace there. It is only when I speak to other women that we slowly find our voices; one woman nervously described waking up to find her toddler feeding from her without her knowledge. In our conversation we each pause before we form the words: almost violent, no consent, a violation. Even as I yearned to feed him, I could simultaneously feel repulsed by the prospect. Where at the beginning there had been absolute, steadfast determination to breastfeed, the conflict within me now grew greater. I was desperate to reclaim some part of myself, but already the shorter, less frequent feeds were like grief.

I found myself torn when he was tired, or sad, or in pain. I knew I had the magic thing that could make everything better and I wanted to give it to him. Even as the faces of those closest to me turned away slightly, as a faint wrinkle of disgust or discomfort passed across their face that had never been there before. Whatever kind of statement my unashamed breastfeeding made when my baby was a newborn was being read as a different kind of statement now.

The truth was, I didn't know how to stop and I wasn't sure I wanted to. I'd already been urged to night-wean by my partner and mum as they saw what I could not see in the mirror: an absolutely broken woman. In the weeks leading up to starting a new part-time job my son had begun waking more and more during the night and nursing was the only thing that would settle him. He moved back into my bed and was soon waking every forty-five minutes. It was a bind; withhold milk and lose sleep as he cried and wailed for hours, or just keep going until somehow it resolved itself? I'd already tried sleeping on the sofa, but the anguished screams as my partner tried to soothe our son were more than I could bear.

So we night-weaned using a method women have used

for centuries: abrupt absence. Children fed by their birth
mothers would be removed to stay with grandparents, or
the mother would stay elsewhere while the father stayed
with the infant. And so, without warning, my mum and my
husband sent me to a hotel for two nights. I put my son
to bed, packed a small bag, and cried all the way to the
bus stop. Halfway across London, the tears stopped and my
shoulders relaxed. By the time I was at the budget hotel I
had acquired wine and snacks and, soon after, I luxuriated
in solitude and sleep. At home, my baby woke up and cried.
For a while. And then he slept through two nights, in bed
beside my partner. The night-time spell was broken, and I
started to gather the shards of my sanity.

But weaning altogether?

In the end the decision was not mine to make. He lost
interest. Our last feed was in February 2020, when he was
eighteen months old and I turned thirty-seven. He suckled,
then broke off and looked up at me, smiling his big, toothy
grin, then returned to the nipple and we played this game
together for a while. And then that was it.

Or at least I thought that was it. Anthropologists have
suggested that in the past, children would have remembered
what it felt like to breastfeed. Palaeo nutritional data indicates that prehistorical infants were not completely weaned
until between the ages of two and six. In antiquity, in Mesopotamia, the Levant and Egypt, children were breastfed
until they were two or three. An Egyptian papyrus states,
'When in due time you were born she still carried you on
her neck and for three years she suckled you.'[1] The Quran
recommends breastfeeding until the age of two. Some Baby-
lonian wet-nursing contracts, dating from the early second
millennium BCE, define the contract period as three years.

What memories will my son have of breastfeeding? Two
months after his last feed we were in the bath together,

singing 'Row, Row, Row the Boat' and making waves. For a brief moment he leaned his face towards my breast, mouth open, and I held my breath, wondering what to do. His eyes met mine and he grinned, paused in that moment of movement, and then it was over and he went back to splashing the water. Was that muscle memory? The way that you might hesitate for a second on greeting an old lover?

Later still, my son was two years and four months and we were going to bed after a long day at nursery. As we read books, he asked to lie on Mummy's tummy, pushing up and under my jumper, placing his head on my bare flesh where he had grown. Only this time he pulled my jumper even higher and pointed to my nipples, counting them triumphantly. Then he looked up at me, serious and questioning: 'Milk, Mummy?' I told him, no, the milk is all gone now. His face erupted into a smile as he proudly deduced that it was 'cos I drank it all'. We laughed and I realised: my body will never make that milk again. Even if I have another baby, it will make a different milk for a different person.

Now, more than a year later, he still stuffs his hand down my jumper when he's afraid. And sometimes, when he snuggles in for a bedtime story, I feel the phantom tug at my nipples. Is that sensation from the same rush of oxytocin, the one that eventually made my milk flow? More than a year since I last breastfed, as I lay submerged in the bathtub during yet another alarmingly hot and humid summer's day, it occurred to me to wonder if my body still possessed the power to make milk. I let the question roll around in my head for a while, an academic exercise of weighing up the potential evolutionary advantages to post-weaning lactation and the knowledge that my periods had returned and I had gone through the noticeable hormonal shift caused by cessation of breastfeeding. I had read about women who had induced lactation in themselves using a combination of hormonal therapy and manual stimulation. I knew it was something that some same-sex couples tried. So there, in the bathtub, I gingerly reached for my breast. I squeezed the soft flesh, gently at first and then more firmly, remembering those instructional videos. Thinking about your baby helps the milk flow, they said; so I conjured a vivid memory of my son's mouth latching on to my nipple and the rhythmic tug of his suck. And then, slowly, thick dark yellow liquid appeared, like custard through a sieve. I dabbed at it with my finger, which I then brought to my mouth to taste. For some reason, I expected it to taste sour, like curdled milk left to solidify in an old bottle. But it didn't.

One afternoon much later, I idly picked through some art books in a charity shop. I found one written by one of my former art history lecturers, on the painter and printmaker Mary Cassatt, who was born in Pennsylvania but spent most of her life in France. I was familiar with her work and admired her Japanese-influenced prints, but her paintings had never before grabbed my attention; but as I flicked through the plates of her studies of breastfeeding, I drew a sharp intake of breath, struck by the accuracy of the detail. Her studies of mothers and infants are perhaps the most astute portrayals of the love and bonding, the ambivalence and exhaustion, the longing and the resigned. Cassatt captures all this longing and nostalgia in paint. I immediately sent a photo to a friend, who had also recently weaned her daughter, and she wrote back telling me the image moved her to tears.

Cassatt was an outspoken feminist and a vocal supporter of suffrage, and deplored being stereotyped as a 'woman artist'. She made radical and influential contributions artistically, but was also central to advancing knowledge and patronage of the Impressionist painters in both Europe and

North America. Despite this, she tends now to only appear in the margins of art history. Much of her work exploring woman and child captures moments of mothering *work*: bathing the child, feeding the child, washing the child's toes. There is an obvious physical labour involved in these tasks, as any reader who has ever filled a paddling pool with a bucket or wiped up encrusted cereal will know. As art historian Griselda Pollock writes: 'Cassatt does not produce modernist madonnas. No madonna is shown working at her job.'[2] Yet, while breastfeeding is a job, it is also many other things. It is this something else, this in-between that I find in Cassatt's 1906 work *Young Mother Nursing Her Child*, now in the Art Institute in Chicago. The deep eye contact, the baby's fingers exploring the mother's mouth, the mother's hand clutching an errant foot. The naked baby wriggles, a leg kicks at the woman's thigh.

It would be a mistake to read these works as autobiographical. In any case, Cassatt never had children. Instead, the more I look at her nursing images, the more I see her paintings as love letters from child to mother, the former entirely relaxed and comfortable as themselves, enveloped within their mother's safe embrace. Vivid memories of maternal nurturing sustained Louise Bourgeois, who recalled, 'I felt that what I represented was the true naked body of the child with the mother. I can still feel her body and her love.'[3]

Cassatt's infants remind me that I all too often forget the receiver of milk: the child. 'To wean' is a transitive verb; it moves us from one place to another. The term has its roots in *wenian*, Old English for 'to accustom; habituate; prepare; train; make fit'. What are we training them for with this milk? I trace those etymological branches back further to Proto-Indo-European and *wenh*, which means 'to strive for; wish; love'. This is what my milk is – something for the present, yes, but also for the future. Remember this. And maybe, in some bat-squeak echo from decades past, we do remember. The hand that fed us. What I see in Cassatt's work is the memory of childhood: I remember what it felt like to be held by you.

But the dyad relationship is also characterised by forgetting. Now, just a year on – or is it two years? – the knuckle-biting pain of nursing has receded. I can write about it, but I can't *feel* it any more. I don't even recognise the woman I'm writing about, she who was so fragile and afraid. But that tiny hand that patted my rib the first day he nursed continues with its rhythmic, reassuring tap. His hand still pats mine while I read him a story, as he strokes my cheek while I lie next to him when he can't sleep. That pat tells me it's OK. It tells me, *Mummy, I am slowly growing up and away from you and it's not all on you any more.*

Milk is natural. But our bodies don't exist in isolation. Our bodies and our lives are subject to various 'unnatural' pressures: capitalism, patriarchy, racism and so on. This is especially urgent given the move towards conservatism, where women's rights are threatened on a seemingly never-ending basis. Breastfeeding can often be beautiful, but that beauty needs to be held and sustained by more than just the breastfeeding parent. That parent needs help as they are battered by the storm of social, moral and cultural expectations.

I think about this as I watch my son gliding ahead on his scooter, long body, strong legs, confident. He slices through a puddle. It's deeper than he'd expected, and he whoops with glee, pressing his wellied foot into the pavement with force. He glides round a corner and is, briefly, out of sight. There he goes, moving forward in the world, further and further ahead of me, away from me. He loves unicorns, horses, trains and milk. He'd drink milk all day if allowed.

I wonder if this unquenchable thirst comes from a lack at the very beginning, the need to make sure he is never without again. But as I watch him propelling himself forward, I see that thirst again. I see it in everything he does.

He drags the rubber toe of his boot along the ground and comes to a stop. He turns round to smile at me. My heart swells, pushing into my breastbone. 'Come,' he calls. So I follow. Milk was just the beginning.

NOTES

Introduction

1 R. Jakobson, 'Why "Mama" and "Papa"?', in *Readings in Modern Linguistics: An Anthology* (De Gruyter Mouton, 2019), pp. 313–20.

2 Andrea O'Reilly, 'Matricentric Feminism: A Feminism for Mothers', in *Journal of the Motherhood Initiative*, Vol 10, No 1–2 (2019), pp. 13–15.

3 M. Erica Couto-Ferreira, 'Being Mothers or Acting (like) Mothers? Constructing Motherhood in Ancient Mesopotamia', in *Women in Antiquity: Real Women across the Ancient World*, eds Stephanie Lynn Budin and Jean Macintosh Turfa (London: Routledge, 2016).

4 Nigel C. Rollins and others, 'Why Invest, and What It Will Take to Improve Breastfeeding Practices?', *The Lancet*, 387.10017 (2016), 491–504.

5 Gill Thomson, Katherine Ebisch-Burton, and Renee Flacking, 'Shame If You Do – Shame If You Don't: Women's Experiences of Infant Feeding', *Maternal & Child Nutrition*, 11.1 (2015), 33–46.

6 Hallie J. Kintner, 'Trends and Regional Differences in Breastfeeding in Germany From 1871 To 1937', *Journal of Family History*, 10.2 (1985), 163–82.

7 John Knodel and Etienne Van de Walle, 'Breast Feeding, Fertility and Infant Mortality: An Analysis of Some Early German Data.', *Population Studies*, 21.2 (1967), 119.

Chapter 1

1   Pranee Liamputtong, *Childrearing and Infant Care Issues: A Cross-Cultural Perspective* (Nova Publishers, 2007), p. 13.

2   Nirupama Laroia and Deeksha Sharma, 'The Religious and Cultural Bases for Breastfeeding Practices Among the Hindus', in *Breastfeeding Medicine*, (2006), pp. 94–8.

3   Jacques Guillemeau, *Child-Birth or, The Happy Delivery of Vvomen* (London: Printed by Anne Griffin, for Ioyce Norton, and Richard Whitaker, 1635).

4   Victoria Sparey, 'Breastfeeding Mothers and Milk in Shakespeare', *Early Modern Medicine*, 2013.

5   G. Corrington, 'The Milk of Salvation: Redemption by the Mother in Late Antiquity and Early Christianity', *Harvard Theological Review*, 82.4 (1989).

6   Mones Abu-Asab, Hakima Amri, and Marc S. Micozzi, *Avicenna's Medicine: A New Translation of the 11th-Century Canon with Practical Applications for Integrative Health Care* (Healing Arts, 2013), 258.

7   Pascale F. Engelmajer, '"Like a Mother Her Only Child": Mothering in the Pāli Canon', *Open Theology*, 6.1 (2020), 88–103.

8   Valerie Fildes, *Breasts, Bottles, and Babies* (Edinburgh: Edinburgh University Press, 1986), 5.

9   Quoted by Laurence Totelin, 'Of Milk and Honey', *Concoctinghistory*, 2013, https://ancientrecipes.wordpress.com/2013/05/14/of-milk-and-honey [accessed 15 July 2021].

10 Laurence Totelin, 'Of Milk and Honey II', *Concoctinghistory*, 2013, https://ancientrecipes.wordpress.com/2013/05/30/of-milk-and-honey-ii [accessed 15 July 2021].

11 Suśruta and Bhishagratna, *An English Translation of the Sushruta Samhita Based on Original Sanskrit Text*, pp. 433–5.

12 Marylynn Salmon, 'The Cultural Significance of Breastfeeding and Infant Care in Early Modern England and America', *Journal of Social History*, 28.2 (1994), 249

13 Marylynn Salmon, 'The Cultural Significance of Breastfeeding and Infant Care in Early Modern England and America', *Journal of Social History*, 28.2 (1994), 247–69.

14 Sir Astley Paston Cooper, *On the Anatomy of the Breast* (London: Longman, Orme, Green, Brown, and Longmans, 1840).

15 Druin Burch, 'Astley Paston Cooper (1768–1841): Anatomist, Radical and Surgeon', *Journal of the Royal Society of Medicine*, 103.12 (2010), 505–8.

16 Saad S. Al-Shehri and others, 'Breastmilk-Saliva Interactions Boost Innate Immunity by Regulating the Oral Microbiome in Early Infancy', *PLOS ONE*, 10.9 (2015).

17 Katie Hinde and others, 'Cortisol in Mother's Milk across Lactation Reflects Maternal Life History and Predicts Infant Temperament', *Behavioral Ecology*, 26.1 (2014), 269–81.

18 Sir Astley Paston Cooper, *On the Anatomy of the Breast* (London: Longman, Orme, Green, Brown, and Longmans, 1840), 134–6.

19 Alia Heise and Diane Wiessinger, 'Dysphoric Milk Ejection Reflex: A Case Report', *International Breastfeeding Journal*, 6 (2011).

20 Zainab Yate, *When Breastfeeding Sucks* (Pinter & Martin, 2020).

Chapter 2

1 *Yemoja: Gender, Sexuality, and Creativity in the Latina/o and Afro-Atlantic Diasporas*, eds Solimar Otero and Toyin Falola (State University of New York Press, 2013), xviii.

2 Z. S. Strother, 'A Terrifying Mimesis: Problems of Portraiture and Representation in African Sculpture (Congo-Kinshasa)', *Res: Anthropology and Aesthetics*, 65–66 (2015), 128–47.

3 Catharine H. Roehrig, 'Women's Work: Some Occupations of Non-Royal Women as Depicted in Ancient Egyptian Art', in *Mistress of the House, Mistress of Heaven: Women in Ancient Egypt*, eds Anne K. Capel and Glenn E. Markoe (New York: Hudson Hills Press, 1996); Marsha Hill, 'Nursing Women', in *Egyptian Art in the Age of the Pyramids* (New York: Metropolitan Museum of Art, 1999), pp. 393–4.

4 Sharri R. Clark, 'Material Matters: Representation and Materiality of the Harappan Body', *Journal of Archaeological Method and Theory*, 16.3 (2009), 231–61.

5 Dayong Yang, Songming Peng, Mark R. Hartman, Tiffany Gupton-Campolongo, Edward J. Rice, Anna Kathryn Chang, et al., 'Enhanced Transcription and Translation in Clay Hydrogel and Implications for Early Life Evolution', *Scientific Reports*, 3.1 (2013), 3165.

6   G. Corrington, 'The Milk of Salvation: Redemption by the
    Mother in Late Antiquity and Early Christianity.', *Harvard
    Theological Review*, 82.4 (1989), 400.

7   Ally Kateusz, *Mary and Early Christian Women* (Palgrave
    Macmillan, 2019), 29.

8   G. Corrington, 'The Milk of Salvation: Redemption by the
    Mother in Late Antiquity and Early Christianity.', *Harvard
    Theological Review*, 82.4 (1989), 411.

9   K. Knight and others, *Saving Lives, Improving Mothers' Care
    – Lessons Learned to Inform Maternity Care from the UK
    and Ireland Confidential Enquiries into Maternal Deaths and
    Morbidity 2017–19* (Oxford: National Perinatal Epidemi-
    ology Unit, University of Oxford, 2021).

Chapter 3

1   G. E. Bentley, *William Blake: The Critical Heritage* (London:
    Routledge, 1995), 36–7.

2   Magdalena Ohaja and Chinemerem Anyim, 'Rituals and
    Embodied Cultural Practices at the Beginning of Life: African
    Perspectives', *Religions*, 12.11 (2021).

3   E. Hoban, 'We're Safe and Happy Already: Traditional Birth
    Attendants and Safe Motherhood in a Cambodian Rural
    Commune' (unpublished PhD thesis, The University of Mel-
    bourne, 2002).

Chapter 5

1   bell hooks, *Feminist Theory: From Margin to Center* (South
    End Press, 1984), 134–5.

2   Linda M. Blum, 'Mothers, Babies, and Breastfeeding in Late
    Capitalist America: The Shifting Contexts of Feminist The-
    ory', *Feminist Studies*, 19.2 (1993), 291–311.

3   Keren Epstein-Gilboa, 'Breastfeeding Envy: Unresolved Pa-
    triarchal Envy and the Obstruction of Physiologically-Based
    Nursing Patterns', in *Giving Breastmilk: Body Ethics and
    Contemporary Breastfeeding Practices*, eds Rhonda Shaw and
    Alison Bartlett (Toronto: Demeter Press, 2010).

4   Adrienne Rich, *Of Woman Born: Motherhood as an Experi-
    ence and Institution* (New York: Norton, 1986).

5   Andrea O'Reilly, 'Matricentric Feminism: A Feminism for

Mothers', *Journal of the Motherhood Initiative*, 10.1–2 (2019), 22.

6   Pascale F. Engelmajer, '"Like a Mother Her Only Child": Mothering in the Pāli Canon', *Open Theology*, 6.1 (2020), 88–103.

7   Penny Van Esterik, 'Rice And Milk In Thai Buddhism: Symbolic And Social Values Of Basic Food Substances', *Crossroads: An Interdisciplinary Journal of Southeast Asian Studies*, 2.1 (1984), 55.

8   Catherine Hodge Mccoid and Leroy D. Mcdermott, 'Toward Decolonizing Gender', American Anthropologist, 98.2 (1996), 319–26.

Chapter 6

1   Julia Kristeva, *Powers of Horror* (New York: Columbia University Press, 1982), 4.

2   Ros Bramwell, 'An Initial Quantitative Study of the Relationship between Attitudes to Menstruation and Breastfeeding', *Journal of Reproductive and Infant Psychology*, 26.3 (2008), 244–55.

3   Nadia Maria Filippini, *Pregnancy, Delivery, Childbirth. A Gender and Cultural History from Antiquity to the Test Tube in Europe* (Oxon: Routledge, 2021), 12–13.

4   Nadia Maria Filippini, *Pregnancy, Delivery, Childbirth. A Gender and Cultural History from Antiquity to the Test Tube in Europe* (Oxon: Routledge, 2021), 10.

5   Amy Brown, *Why Breastfeeding Grief and Trauma Matter* (Pinter & Martin, 2019).

6   Ariell Ahearn, 'Milk, Female Labor, and Human-Animal Relations in Contemporary Mongolia', in *Socialist and Post-Socialist Mongolia*, eds Simon Wickhamsmith and Phillip P. Marzluf (London: Routledge, 2021).

7   William Stephens, 'Lactile Libations: Mongolian Milk Offerings', *Missiology*, 49.1 (2021), 39–53.

8   Rebecca M. Empson, *Harnessing Fortune: Personhood, Memory and Place in Mongolia* (Oxford University Press, 2011).

9   OECD and World Health Organization, *Health at a Glance: Asia/Pacific 2020: Measuring Progress Towards Universal Health Coverage*, Health at a Glance: Asia/Pacific (OECD, 2020).

Chapter 7

1 Monica Green, *Making Women's Medicine Masculine: The Rise of Male Authority in Pre-Modern Gynaecology* (Oxford: Oxford University Press, 2008).

2 William Cadogan M.D., *An Essay upon Nursing, and the Management of Children, from Their Birth to Three Years of Age*, 3rd edn (London: J. Roberts, 1749).

3 William Buchan, *Domestic Medicine or the Family Physician* (New York: Richard Scott).

4 Hugh Smith, *Letters to Married Women on Nursing and the Management of Children*, 2nd edn (Philadephia: Mathew Carey, 1796), 63.

5 Hugh Smith, *Letters to Married Women on Nursing and the Management of Children*, 2nd edn (Philadephia: Mathew Carey, 1796), 52–3.

6 Nora Doyle, *Maternal Bodies* (University of North Carolina Press, 2018).

7 'Mothers Told "Breast Milk Is Best"', *BBC News*, 17 May 1999 http://news.bbc.co.uk/1/hi/health/345693.stm [accessed 25 November 2021].

8 Matthew D. Mendham, 'Rousseau's Discarded Children: The Panoply of Excuses and the Question of Hypocrisy', *History of European Ideas*, 41.1 (2015), 131–52; William Kessen, 'Rousseau's Children', *Daedalus*, 107.3 (1978), 155–66.

9 Carol Duncan, 'Happy Mothers and Other New Ideas in French Art', *The Art Bulletin*, 55.4 (1973), 582.

10 Jessica Cox, 'The "Most Sacred of Duties": Maternal Ideals and Discourses of Authority in Victorian Breastfeeding Advice', *Journal of Victorian Culture*, 25.2 (2020), 223–39.

11 Marylynn Salmon, 'The Cultural Significance of Breastfeeding and Infant Care in Early Modern England and America', *Journal of Social History*, 28.2 (1994), 247–69.

12 'The Advantages of Maternal Nurture', Ladies' Monthly Museum, 184, quoted in Nora Doyle, *Maternal Bodies* (University of North Carolina Press, 2018), p. 94.

13 Katharina Rowold, 'Modern Mothers, Modern Babies: Breastfeeding and Mother's Milk in Interwar Britain', *Women's History Review*, 28 (2019), 1–20.

14 Ibid.

Chapter 8

1   Robbie Pfeufer Kahn, 'Women and Time in Childbirth and During Lactation', in *Feminist Perspectives on Temporality*, eds Frieda Johles Forman and Caoran Sowton (Oxford: Pergamon Press, 1988), 28.
2   Conway & Young, *Milk Report*, 2019.
3   Robbie Pfeufer Kahn, 'Women and Time in Childbirth and During Lactation', in Feminist Perspectives on Temporality, eds Frieda Johles Forman and Caoran Sowton (Oxford: Pergamon Press, 1988), pp. 20–36; Jay Griffiths, *Pip Pip. A Sideways Look at Time* (London: HarperPress, 2000).

Chapter 9

1   Margarita Sánchez Romero and Rosa López, 'Motherhood and Infancies: Archaeological and Historical Approaches', in *Motherhood and Infancies in the Mediterranean in Antiquity*, 2018, 5.
2   Gérard Coulon, *L'Enfant En Gaule Romaine. Deuxième Édition Entièrement Revue et Augmentée.* (Paris: Errance, Hespérides, 2004), 69.
3   J. Dunne and others, 'Milk of Ruminants in Ceramic Baby Bottles from Prehistoric Child Graves', *Nature*, 574.7777 (2019), 246–48.
4   *The Rock-Art of Eastern North America: Capturing Images and Insight*, eds Carol Diaz-Granados and James Duncan (University Alabama Press, 2010).

Chapter 10

1   Cristina Mazzoni, *She-Wolf. The Story of a Roman Icon* (Cambridge University Press, 2010), 6.
2   Clare Johnson and Jenny Rintoul, 'From Nursing Virgins to Brelfies: The Project of Maternal Femininity', *Journal of Gender Studies*, 28.8 (2019), 918–36.
3   Les Mitchell, *Reading the Animal Text in the Landscape of the Damned* (NISC (Pty) Ltd, 2019), 31.
4   William Cadogan M.D., *An Essay upon Nursing, and the Management of Children, from Their Birth to Three Years of Age*, 3rd edn (London: J. Roberts, 1749).
5   Vivien Jones, 'The Death of Mary Wollstonecraft', *Journal for*

Eighteenth-Century Studies, 20.2 (1997), 187–205.

6   Valerie Fildes, 'The Culture and Biology of Breastfeeding: An Historical Review of Western Europe', in *Breastfeeding: Biocultural Perspectives* (Routledge, 1995), 116.

7   Valerie Fildes, 'The Culture and Biology of Breastfeeding: An Historical Review of Western Europe', in *Breastfeeding: Biocultural Perspectives* (Routledge, 1995), 118.

8   Patricia Stuart-Macadam, 'Breastfeeding in Prehistory', in *Breastfeeding: Biocultural Perspectives*, eds Patricia Stuart-Macadam and Katherine A. Dettwyler (New York: Aldine de Gruyter, 1995), 83.

9   Marylynn Salmon, 'The Cultural Significance of Breastfeeding and Infant Care in Early Modern England and America', *Journal of Social History*, 28.2 (1994), 256.

10 Rima D. Apple, '"To Be Used Only Under The Direction Of A Physician": Commercial Infant Feeding And Medical Practice, 1870–1940', *Bulletin of the History of Medicine*, 54.3 (1980), 402–17.

11 Gerard Hastings and others, 'Selling Second Best: How Infant Formula Marketing Works', *Globalization and Health*, 16.1 (2020), 77.

12 Ibid.

13 Linda M. Blum, 'Mothers, Babies, and Breastfeeding in Late Capitalist America: The Shifting Contexts of Feminist Theory', *Feminist Studies*, 19.2 (1993), 301.

14 AFP, 'Cambodia Bans Export of Human Breast Milk after US Operation Raises Concern', *Guardian*, 28 March 2017, https://www.theguardian.com/world/2017/mar/28/cambodia-breast-milk-us-export-ambrosia-labs [accessed 27 April 2021].

15 Wong, Tessa, 'Cambodia Breast Milk: The Debate over Mothers Selling Milk', *BBC News*, 29 March 2017, https://www.bbc.com/news/world-asia-39414820 [accessed 20 June 2021].

Chapter 11

1   Bernice Hausman, 'The Feminist Politics of Breastfeeding', *Australian Feminist Studies*, 19.45 (2004), 274.

2   Rebecca Kukla, 'Ethics and Ideology in Breastfeeding Advocacy Campaigns', *Hypatia*, 21.1 (2006), 157–80.

3 Tara Cassidy, 'Breastfeeding Mothers Protest Alleged Treatment of Mother by Shopping Centre Staff', *ABC News*, 28 May 2021, https://www.abc.net.au/news/2021-05-28/breastfeeding-protest-at-gold-coast-pacific-fair/100172194 [accessed 3 November 2021]; Jessica Campisi and Saeed Ahmed, '2 Moms Were Scolded for Breastfeeding at a Pool. More than a Dozen Others Joined Them in Protest', *CNN*, https://www.cnn.com/2018/07/24/health/breastfeeding-moms-pool-protest-trnd/index.html [accessed 3 November 2021]; Frieze News Desk, 'Breastfeeding Mothers Protest at Mexico City's Museum of Modern Art', *Frieze*, 2019, https://www.frieze.com/article/breastfeeding-mothers-protest-mexico-citys-museum-modern-art [accessed 3 November 2021].

4 Aleksandra Maria Męcińska, 'Social Struggles Over Breastfeeding: How Lactivism Reshapes Knowledge, Meanings, And Practices Of Breastfeeding' (unpublished PhD thesis, Lancaster University, 2017), 8.

5 Mark Sweney, 'Mums Furious as Facebook Removes Breastfeeding Photos', *Guardian*, 30 December 2008, section Technology, https://www.theguardian.com/media/2008/dec/30/facebook-breastfeeding-ban [accessed 27 November 2021].

6 Amy Brown, 'Are We Really Still Talking about a Woman's Right to Breastfeed in Public?', UNICEF, 2018, https://www.unicef.org.uk/babyfriendly/still-talking-about-a-womans-right-to-breastfeed-in-public [accessed 12 July 2021].

7 R. Buller, 'Performing the Breastfeeding Body: Lactivism and Art Interventions', *Studies in the Maternal*, 8.2 (2016) 14; Wendy Widom, 'Facebook & Instagram Are Censoring Motherhood, Says 4th Trimester Bodies Project', *CBS News Chicago*, 30 July 2014, https://www.cbsnews.com/chicago/news/4th-trimester-bodies-project-facebook-instagram [accessed 27 November 2021].

8 Jonathan Blake, 'Instagram Allows Breastfeeding and Post-Op Scars in New Guidelines', *BBC News*, 16 April 2015, section Newsbeat, https://www.bbc.com/news/newsbeat-32340412 [accessed 27 November 2021].

9 Aimee Dawson, 'Facebook Censors 30,000 Year-Old Venus of Willendorf as "Pornographic"', *The Art Newspaper*, 2018,

https://www.theartnewspaper.com/2018/02/27/facebook-censors-30000-year-old-venus-of-willendorf-as-pornographic [accessed 27 November 2021].

10 'Facebook Apologizes for Censoring Prehistoric Figurine "Venus of Willendorf"', DW.COM, 1 March 2018, https://www.dw.com/en/facebook-apologizes-for-censoring-prehistoric-figurine-venus-of-willendorf/a-42780200 [accessed 27 November 2021].

11 Rebecca Kukla, 'Ethics and Ideology in Breastfeeding Advocacy Campaigns', *Hypatia*, 21.1 (2006), 157–80.

12 Ashifa Kassam, 'Breastfeeding as a Trans Dad: "A Baby Doesn't Know What Your Pronouns Are"', *Guardian*, 20 June 2016, section Society, https://www.theguardian.com/society/2016/jun/20/transgender-dad-breastfeeding-pregnancy-trevor-macdonald [accessed 27 September 2021]; Trevor MacDonald, *Where's the Mother?: Stories from a Transgender Dad* (Trans Canada Press, 2016).

13 Josh Tapper, 'La Leche League Canada Rejects Breastfeeding Dad's Bid to Become Lactation Coach', *Toronto Star*, 19 August 2012, section Canada, https://www.thestar.com/news/canada/2012/08/19/la_leche_league_canada_rejects_breastfeeding_dads_bid_to_become_lactation_coach.html [accessed 20 November 2021].

14 Josh Tapper, 'Transgender Man Can Be Breastfeeding Coach', *Toronto Star*, 25 April 2014, section Health & Wellness, https://www.thestar.com/life/health_wellness/2014/04/25/transgender_man_can_be_breastfeeding_coach.html [accessed 20 November 2021].

15 Trevor MacDonald and others, 'Transmasculine Individuals' Experiences with Lactation, Chestfeeding, and Gender Identity: A Qualitative Study', *BMC Pregnancy and Childbirth*, 16.1 (2016).

16 Buchi Emecheta, *The Joys of Motherhood* (Heinemann, 1979), 34.

17 Theresa Garner, 'Breastfeeding Poster Dropped', *NZ Herald*, 2003, https://www.nzherald.co.nz/nz/breastfeeding-poster-dropped/NZJSQEG5Z6KILCT6LF5EM2T7GA [accessed 20 October 2021].

18 Nadja Sayej, 'Cindy Sherman and Catherine Opie Make a Strangely Charming Cameo in Jewelry Together', *W Magazine*,

2019, https://www.wmagazine.com/story/cindy-sherman-catherine-opie-cameo-lizworks-jewelry [accessed 20 October 2021].

Chapter 12

1 Linda M. Blum, 'Mothers, Babies, and Breastfeeding in Late Capitalist America: The Shifting Contexts of Feminist Theory', *Feminist Studies*, 19.2 (1993), 291–311.
2 Alicia Suskin Ostriker, 'Paragraphs', in *The Mother/Child Papers* (University of Pittsburgh Press, 2009).
3 Alicia Suskin Ostriker, 'Letter to M.', in *The Mother/Child Papers* (University of Pittsburgh Press, 2009), 33.
4 Quoted in Nora Doyle, *Maternal Bodies* (University of North Carolina Press, 2018), 105.
5 Mears, Martha, *The Pupil of Nature; or Candid Advice to the Fair Sex*, (London, 1797), 140.
6 Stretzer, Thomas, *A New Description of Merryland: Containing, a Topographical, Geographical, and Natural History of That Country*, (London: E. Curll, 1742), 37.
7 Thomas Raynalde, *The Birth of Mankind: Otherwise Named, The Woman's Book : Newly Set Forth, Corrected, and Augmented : Whose Contents Ye May Read in the Table of the Book, and Most Plainly in the Prologue / [Eucharius Rösslin] ; [Revised and Augmented] by Thomas Reynalde, Physician, 1560*, ed. Elaine Hobby (Ashgate, 2009).
8 Clare Johnson and Jenny Rintoul, 'From Nursing Virgins to Brelfies: The Project of Maternal Femininity', *Journal of Gender Studies*, 28.8 (2019), 918–36.
9 James Nelson, *An essay on the government of children, under three general heads; viz. health, manners and education*, (London: R.& J. Dodsley, et al., 1753), 46–7.
10 Randolph Trumbach, *The Rise of the Egalitarian Family: Aristocratic Kinship and Domestic Relations in Eighteenth-Century England*, (New York: Academic Press, Inc., 1978) 2201–203.
11 James Nelson, *An essay on the government of children, under three general heads; viz. health, manners and education*, (London: R.& J. Dodsley, et al., 1753), 48.
12 Mrs Seba Smith, 'Anxious Mothers', *The Mother's Assistant and Young Lady's Friend 2, No 12*, (1842), 265–266.

13 Ruth Perry, 'Colonizing the Breast: Sexuality and Maternity in Eighteenth-Century England', *Journal of the History of Sexuality*, 2.2 (1991), 213.

14 Lisa Algazi Marcus, '"Mastomania" Breastfeeding and the Circulation of Desire in Nineteenth-Century France', *Journal of the Motherhood Initiative for Research and Community Involvement*, 7.2 (2017).

15 Iris Marion Young, 'Breasted Experience', in *Throwing Like a Girl and Other Essays in Feminist Philosophy and Social Theory* (Indiana University Press, 1990), pp. 189–209.

16 Iris Marion Young, 'Throwing Like a Girl: A Phenomenology of Feminine Body Comportment, Motility and Spatiality', in *Throwing Like a Girl and Other Essays in Feminist Philosophy and Social Theory* (Indiana University Press, 1990), 199.

17 Fiona Giles, 'The Uses Of Pleasure: Reconfiguring Lactation, Sexuality and Mothering', in *Theorising and Representing Maternal Realities*, eds Marie Porter and Julie Kelso (Cambridge Scholars Publishing, 2008), 21.

18 Adrienne Rich, *Of Woman Born: Motherhood as an Experience and Institution* (New York: Norton, 1986).

19 Jennifer West, 'White Columns', Frieze, 2008, https://web.archive.org/web/20100608093758/http://www.frieze.com/issue/review/jennifer_west [accessed 9 May 2021].

20 Andrea Liss, *Feminist Art and the Maternal* (University of Minnesota Press, 2009), 75.

21 Andrea Liss, *Feminist Art and the Maternal* (University of Minnesota Press, 2009), 76.

22 R. Buller, 'Performing the Breastfeeding Body: Lactivism and Art Interventions', *Studies in the Maternal*, 8.2 (2016), 14.

23 Micol Hebron, 'Reviews: Separation Anxiety', *Art Pulse* http://artpulsemagazine.com/separation-anxiety [accessed 7 November 2021].

Chapter 13

1 Jon Filson, 'Taste Test', *Toronto Star*, 14 July 2006.

2 Penny Van Esterik, 'Breast-Feeding as Food Work', in *Food and Culture*, eds Penny Van Esterik, Caroline Counihan, and Alice Julier (Routledge, 2013).

3 Barry S. Hewlett and Steve Winn, 'Allomaternal Nursing in Humans', *Current Anthropology*, 55.2 (2014), 200–229.

4   Avner Giladi, *Infants, Parents and Wet Nurses: Medieval Islamic Views on Breastfeeding and Their Social Implications* (Leiden: Brill, 1999), 21–31.

Chapter 14

1   Hayden Herrera, *Frida* (London: Bloomsbury, 2003), 10.
2   Lucy Ann Havard, 'Kahlo, Mexicanidad and Máscaras: The Search for Identity in Postcolonial Mexico', *Romance Studies*, 24.3 (2006), 246.
3   Carolyn. E. Tate, *Reconsidering Olmec Visual Culture The Unborn, Women, and Creation* (University of Texas Press, 2012).
4   Tina Kinsella, 'Querying and Queering the Virgin: Iconography and Iconoclasticism in the Art of Frida Kahlo', *Tina Kinsella*, 2011, https://tinakinsella.wordpress.com/72-2 [accessed 6 August 2021].
5   George D. Sussman, 'The Wet-Nursing Business in Nineteenth-Century France', *French Historical Studies*, 9.2 (1975), 304–28.
6   George D. Sussman, 'The Wet-Nursing Business in Nineteenth-Century France', *French Historical Studies*, 9.2 (1975), 309.
7   Carol Duncan, 'Happy Mothers and Other New Ideas in French Art', *The Art Bulletin*, 55.4 (1973), 570–83.
8   Sir Astley Paston Cooper, *On the Anatomy of the Breast* (London: Longman, Orme, Green, Brown, and Longmans, 1840), 143.
9   Catharine H. Roehrig, 'Women's Work: Some Occupations of Non-Royal Women as Depicted in Ancient Egyptian Art', in *Mistress of the House, Mistress of Heaven: Women in Ancient Egypt*, eds Anne K. Capel and Glenn E. Markoe (New York: Hudson Hills Press, 1996).
10 Gayatri Chakravorty Spivak, 'Introduction', in *Breast Stories* (New York: Seagull, 2018), vii.
11 Jennifer L. Morgan, '"Some Could Suckle over Their Shoulder": Male Travelers, Female Bodies, and the Gendering of Racial Ideology, 1500–1770', *The William and Mary Quarterly*, 54.1 (1997), 167–92.
12 Emily West and Emily Knight, 'Mothers' Milk: Slavery, Wet-Nursing, and Black and White Women in the Antebellum South', *Journal of Southern History*, 83 (2017), 39.

13 Ibid., 50.

Chapter 15

1   Bernard J. Davis, 'Migrant Mother: Dorothea Lange and the Truth of Photography', *Los Angeles Review of Books*, 2020, https://lareviewofbooks.org/article/migrant-mother-dorothea-lange-truth-photography [accessed 9 May 2021].
2   Marta Zarzycka, *Gendered Tropes in War Photography: Mothers, Mourners, Soldiers* (New York: Routledge, 2017).
3   Nora Doyle, *Maternal Bodies* (University of North Carolina Press, 2018).
4   Bernard J. Davis, 'Migrant Mother: Dorothea Lange and the Truth of Photography', *Los Angeles Review of Books*, 2020, https://lareviewofbooks.org/article/migrant-mother-dorothea-lange-truth-photography [accessed 9 May 2021].
5   Valerius Maximus, *Memorable Words and Deeds*, trans. Henry John Walker (Indianapolis, 2004), Vol 4 ext. 1, 180.
6   J. Vanessa Lyon, 'Full of Grace: Lactation, Expression and "Colorito" Painting in Some Early Works by Rubens', in *Medieval and Renaissance Lactations*, ed. Jutta Gisela Sperling (Routledge, 2013), 258.
7   Linda M. Blum, 'Mothers, Babies, and Breastfeeding in Late Capitalist America: The Shifting Contexts of Feminist Theory', *Feminist Studies*, 19.2 (1993), 291–311.

Chapter 16

1   Fiona Giles, '"Relational, and Strange": A Preliminary Foray into a Project to Queer Breastfeeding', *Australian Feminist Studies*, 19.45 (2004).
2   M. Walter, 'The Folklore of Breastfeeding', *Bulletin of the New York Academy of Medicine*, 51.7 (1975), 870–76.
3   Nadia Maria Filippini, *Pregnancy, Delivery, Childbirth. A Gender and Cultural History from Antiquity to the Test Tube in Europe* (Oxon: Routledge, 2021), 83–5.
4   Aleksandra Maria Męcińska, 'Social Struggles Over Breastfeeding: How Lactivism Reshapes Knowledge, Meanings, And Practices Of Breastfeeding' (unpublished PhD thesis, Lancaster University, 2017), 71–2.
5   Interview with Zainab Yate, 2021.

6 Donald L. Swearer, 'Hypostasizing the Buddha: Buddha Image Consecration in Northern Thailand', *History of Religions*, Vol 34, No 3, 1995, pp. 263–80.

Epilogue

1 Patricia Stuart-Macadam, 'Breastfeeding in Prehistory', in *Breastfeeding: Biocultural Perspectives*, eds Patricia Stuart-Macadam and Katherine A. Dettwyler (New York: Aldine de Gruyter, 1995), 82–3.

2 Griselda Pollock, *Mary Cassatt: Painter of Modern Women* (London: Thames and Hudson, 1998), 191.

3 Deborah Wye, *Louise Bourgeois* (New York: Museum of Modern Art, 1982), 15.

BIBLIOGRAPHY

Abu-Asab, Mones, Hakima Amri, and Marc S. Micozzi, *Avicenna's Medicine: A New Translation of the 11th-Century Canon with Practical Applications for Integrative Health Care* (Healing Arts, 2013)

AFP, 'Cambodia Bans Export of Human Breast Milk after US Operation Raises Concern', *Guardian*, 28 March 2017, https://www.theguardian.com/world/2017/mar/28/cambodia-breast-milk-us-export-ambrosia-labs [accessed 27 April 2021]

Ahearn, Ariell, 'Milk, Female Labor, and Human-Animal Relations in Contemporary Mongolia', in *Socialist and Post-Socialist Mongolia*, eds Simon Wickhamsmith and Phillip P. Marzluf (London: Routledge, 2021)

Algazi Marcus, Lisa, '"Mastomania" Breastfeeding and the Circulation of Desire in Nineteenth-Century France', *Journal of the Motherhood Initiative for Research and Community Involvement*, 7.2 (2017)

Al-Shehri, Saad S., Christine L. Knox, Helen G. Liley, David M. Cowley, John R. Wright, Michael G. Henman, and others, 'Breastmilk–Saliva Interactions Boost Innate Immunity by Regulating the Oral Microbiome in Early Infancy', *PLOS ONE*, 10.9 (2015)

Amir, Lisa H., 'Breastfeeding in Public: "You Can Do It?"', *International Breastfeeding Journal*, 9 (2014)

Andaya, Barbara Watson, 'Localising the Universal: Women, Motherhood and the Appeal of Early Theravāda Buddhism', *Journal of Southeast Asian Studies*, 33.1 (2002), 1–30

Apple, Rima D., *Mothers and Medicine: Social History of Infant Feeding, 1890–1950* (University of Wisconsin Press, 1988)

———, '"To Be Used Only Under The Direction Of A Physician":

Commercial Infant Feeding And Medical Practice, 1870–1940', Bulletin of the History of Medicine, 54.3 (1980), 402–17

Arnold-Baker, Claire, 'How Becoming a Mother Involves a Confrontation with Existence: An Existential-Phenomenological Exploration of the Experience of Early Motherhood', 2015

——, 'Introduction: The Existential Crisis of Motherhood', in The Existential Crisis of Motherhood, ed. Claire Arnold-Baker (Cham: Springer International Publishing, 2020), pp. 3–16

Aronson, Joshua, Diana Burgess, Sean M. Phelan, and Lindsay Juarez, 'Unhealthy Interactions: The Role of Stereotype Threat in Health Disparities', American Journal of Public Health, 103.1 (2013), 50–6

Badinter, Elisabeth, The Myth of Motherhood: A Historical View of the Maternal Instinct, trans. Roger DeGaris (Souvenir Press, 1981)

Bakar, Faima, 'Breastfeeding Woman Protests and Advocates for Justice for Black Mums', Metro, 2020, https://metro.co.uk/2020/06/08/breastfeeding-woman-protest-children-advocates-justice-black-mums-12820008 [accessed 3 November 2021]

Bal, Mieke, Louise Bourgeois' Spider: The Architecture of Art-Writing (Chicago: University of Chicago Press, 2001)

Ballard, Olivia, and Ardythe L. Morrow, 'Human Milk Composition: Nutrients and Bioactive Factors', Pediatric Clinics of North America, 60.1 (2013), 49–74

Barolsky, Paul, 'Raphael and Breastfeeding', Source: Notes in the History of Art, 34.1 (2014), 16–17

Bauer, Doron, 'Milk As Templar Apologetics In The St. Bernard Of Clairvaux Altarpiece From Majorca', Studies in Iconography, 36 (2015), 79–98

Bentley, G. E., William Blake: The Critical Heritage (London: Routledge, 1995)

Benton, Adia, 'Risky Business: Race, Nonequivalence and the Humanitarian Politics of Life', Visual Anthropology, 29.2 (2016), 187–203

Betterton, Rosemary, 'Louise Bourgeois, Ageing, and Maternal Bodies', Feminist Review, 93.1 (2009), 27–45

Blackall, Molly, '"Stop the Breast Pest": MP's "Horror" at Being Photographed While Breastfeeding', Guardian, 2021 http://www.theguardian.com/lifeandstyle/2021/may/01/

labour-mp-stella-creasy-horror-photographed-while-breastfeeding-prompts-campaign [accessed 20 July 2021]

Blake, Jonathan, 'Instagram Allows Breastfeeding and Post-Op Scars in New Guidelines', *BBC News*, 16 April 2015, section Newsbeat, https://www.bbc.com/news/newsbeat-32340412 [accessed 27 November 2021]

Bloom, Allan, 'The Education of Democratic Man: Emile', *Daedalus*, 107.3 (1978), 135–53

Blum, Linda M., 'Mothers, Babies, and Breastfeeding in Late Capitalist America: The Shifting Contexts of Feminist Theory', *Feminist Studies*, 19.2 (1993), 291–311

Bode, Lars, Mark McGuire, Juan M. Rodriguez, Donna T. Geddes, Foteini Hassiotou, Peter E. Hartmann, and others, 'It's Alive: Microbes and Cells in Human Milk and Their Potential Benefits to Mother and Infant', *Advances in Nutrition* (Bethesda, Md.), 5.5 (2014), 571–73

Bourgeois, Louise, *Midwife to the Queen of France: Diverse Observations*, trans. Stephanie O'Hara and Alison Klairmont Lingo (Toronto: Iter Press, 2017)

Boursier, Louise Bourgeois, *He Serious and Most Choice Secrets of Madame Louyse Bourgioes [sic] . . . Which She Left to Her Daughter as a Guide for Her, Etc* (London, 1680)

Bradley, Keith R., 'Sexual Regulations in Wet-Nursing Contracts from Roman Egypt', *Klio*, 62.62 (1980), 321–26

Brady, June Pauline, 'Marketing Breast Milk Substitutes: Problems and Perils throughout the World', *Archives of Disease in Childhood*, 97.6 (2012), 529

Bramwell, Ros, 'An Initial Quantitative Study of the Relationship between Attitudes to Menstruation and Breastfeeding', *Journal of Reproductive and Infant Psychology*, 26.3 (2008), 244–55

———, 'Blood and Milk: Constructions of Female Bodily Fluids in Western Society', *Women & Health*, 34.4 (2001), 85–96

Breastfeeding Prevalence at 6 to 8 Weeks after Birth (Experimental Statistics) Annual Data Statistical Commentary 2019 to 2020 (Public Health England, February 2021)

Britton, K., E. McManus-Fry, A. Cameron, P. Duffy, E. Masson-MacLean, O. Czére, and others, 'Isotopes and New Norms: Investigating the Emergence of Early Modern U.K. Breastfeeding Practices at St. Nicholas Kirk, Aberdeen', *International Journal of Osteoarchaeology*, 28.5 (2018), 510–22

Brown, A., 'Breastfeeding as a Public Health Responsibility: A Review of the Evidence', *Journal of Human Nutrition and Dietetics*, 30.6 (2017), 759–70

Brown, Amy, 'Are We Really Still Talking about a Woman's Right to Breastfeed in Public?', UNICEF, 2018, https://www.unicef.org.uk/babyfriendly/still-talking-about-a-womans-right-to-breastfeed-in-public [accessed 12 July 2021]

——, *Why Breastfeeding Grief and Trauma Matter* (Pinter & Martin, 2019)

Brown, Amy, and Sue Jordan, 'Impact of Birth Complications on Breastfeeding Duration: An Internet Survey', *Journal of Advanced Nursing*, 69.4 (2013), 828–39

Brown, Amy, J. Rance, and L. Warren, 'Body Image Concerns during Pregnancy Are Associated with a Shorter Breast Feeding Duration', *Midwifery*, 31.1 (2015), 80–89

Brown, Amy, Jaynie Rance, and Paul Bennett, 'Understanding the Relationship between Breastfeeding and Postnatal Depression: The Role of Pain and Physical Difficulties', *Journal of Advanced Nursing*, 72.2 (2016), 273–82

Brown, Amy, Peter Raynor, and Michelle Lee, 'Young Mothers Who Choose to Breast Feed: The Importance of Being Part of a Supportive Breast-Feeding Community', *Midwifery*, 27.1 (2011), 53–59

Buchan, William, *Advice to Mothers; on the Subject of Their Own Health; and of the Means of Promoting the Health, Strength, and Beauty of Their Offspring.* (London: Cadell and Davies, 1803)

Buller, R., 'Performing the Breastfeeding Body: Lactivism and Art Interventions', *Studies in the Maternal*, 8.2 (2016)

Burch, Druin, 'Astley Paston Cooper (1768–1841): Anatomist, Radical and Surgeon', *Journal of the Royal Society of Medicine*, 103.12 (2010), 505–8

Cadogan, William, M.D., *An Essay upon Nursing, and the Management of Children, from Their Birth to Three Years of Age.*, 3rd edn (London: J. Roberts, 1749)

Cassidy, T.M., 'Mothers, Milk and Money: Maternal Corporeal Generosity, Social Psychological Trust, and Value in Human Milk Exchange', *Journal of the Motherhood Initiative for Research and Community Involvement*, 3.1 (2012)

Cassidy, Tara, 'Breastfeeding Mothers Protest Alleged Treatment of

Mother by Shopping Centre Staff', *ABC News*, 28 May 2021, https://www.abc.net.au/news/2021-05-28/breastfeeding-protest-at-gold-coast-pacific-fair/100172194   [accessed   3 November 2021]

Chamberlayne, T., *The Compleat Midwifes Practice, in the Most Weighty and High Concernments of the Birth of Man. Containing Perfect Rules for Midwifes and Nurses, as Also for Women in Their Conception, Bearing, and Nursing of Children: From the Experience Not Onely of Our English, but Also the Most Accomplisht and Absolute Practicers among the French, Spanish, Italian, and Other Nations. A Work so Plain, That the Weakest Capacity May Easily Attain the Knowledge of the Whole Art. With Instructions of the Midwife to the Queen of France (given to Her Daughter a Little before Her Death) Touching the Practice of the Said Art. / Published with the Approbation and Good Liking of Sundry the Most Knowing Professors of Midwifery Now Living in the City of London, and Other Places. Illustrated with Severall Cuts in Brass* (London: Printed for Nathaniel Brooke at the Angell in Cornhill, 1656)

Chavasse, Pye Henry, *Advice to Mothers on the Management of Their Offspring*, 3rd edn (London: Longman, Brown, Green and Longmans, 18)

———, *Advice to Wives on the Management of Themselves, during the Periods of Pregnancy, Labour, and Suckling . . .* , 2nd edn (London: Longman & Co, 1843)

Clark, Gillian, *Correspondence of the Foundling Hospital Inspectors in Berkshire 1757–68* (Berkshire Record Society, 1994), I

Clark, Harri R., 'Representing the Indus Body: Sex, Gender, Sexuality, and the Anthropomorphic Terracotta Figurines from Harappa', *Asian Perspectives*, 42, 2003

Clark, Sharri R., 'Material Matters: Representation and Materiality of the Harappan Body', *Journal of Archaeological Method and Theory*, 16.3 (2009), 231–61

Cook, Katsi, 'Cook: Women Are the First Environment', *Indian Country Today*, 23 December 2003, https://indiancountrytoday.com/archive/cook-women-are-the-first-environment#:~:text=In%20the%20Mohawk%20language%2C%20one,is%20full%20of%20ecological%20context [accessed 10 October 2021]

Cooper, Sir Astley Paston, *On the Anatomy of the Breast* (London: Longman, Orme, Green, Brown, and Longmans, 1840)

Cornell University, 'Clay May Have Been Birthplace of Life on Earth, New Study Suggests', ScienceDaily, 2013, https://www.sciencedaily.com/releases/2013/11/131105132027.htm [accessed 9 November 2021]

Corrington, G., 'The Milk of Salvation: Redemption by the Mother in Late Antiquity and Early Christianity', *Harvard Theological Review*, 82.4 (1989)

Coulon, Gérard, *L'Enfant En Gaule Romaine: Deuxième Édition Entièrement Revue et Augmentée* (Paris: Errance, Hespérides, 2004)

Couto-Ferreira, M. Erica, 'Being Mothers or Acting (like) Mothers? Constructing Motherhood in Ancient Mesopotamia', in *Women in Antiquity: Real Women across the Ancient World*, eds Stephanie Lynn Budin and Jean Macintosh Turfa (London: Routledge, 2016)

Cox, Jessica, 'The "Most Sacred of Duties": Maternal Ideals and Discourses of Authority in Victorian Breastfeeding Advice', *Journal of Victorian Culture*, 25.2 (2020), 223–39

Davis, Bernard J., 'Migrant Mother: Dorothea Lange and the Truth of Photography', *Los Angeles Review of Books*, 2020, https://lareviewofbooks.org/article/migrant-mother-dorothea-lange-truth-photography [accessed 9 May 2021]

Dawson, Aimee, 'Facebook Censors 30,000 Year-Old Venus of Willendorf as "Pornographic"', *The Art Newspaper*, 2018, https://www.theartnewspaper.com/2018/02/27/facebook-censors-30000-year-old-venus-of-willendorf-as-pornographic [accessed 27 November 2021]

Desk, Frieze News, 'Breastfeeding Mothers Protest at Mexico City's Museum of Modern Art', *Frieze*, 2019, https://www.frieze.com/article/breastfeeding-mothers-protest-mexico-citys-museum-modern-art [accessed 3 November 2021]

DW.COM, 'Facebook Apologizes for Censoring Prehistoric Figurine "Venus of Willendorf"', 1 March 2018, https://www.dw.com/en/facebook-apologizes-for-censoring-prehistoric-figurine-venus-of-willendorf/a-42780200 [accessed 27 November 2021].

Devi, Mahasweta, *Breast Stories*, trans. Gayatri Chakravorty Spivak (London: Seagull, 2018)

Diaz-Granados, Carol, and James Duncan, eds, *The Rock-Art of Eastern North America: Capturing Images and Insight* (University Alabama Press, 2010)

Dowling, Sally, and Amy Brown, 'An Exploration of the Experiences of Mothers Who Breastfeed Long-Term: What Are the Issues and Why Does It Matter?', *Breastfeeding Medicine*, 8.1 (2013), 45–52

Doyle, Nora, *Maternal Bodies* (University of North Carolina Press, 2018)

Duncan, Carol, 'Happy Mothers and Other New Ideas in French Art', *The Art Bulletin*, 55.4 (1973), 570–83

Dunn, P.M., 'Louise Bourgeois (1563–1636): Royal Midwife of France', *Archives of Disease in Childhood – Fetal and Neonatal Edition*, 89 (2004), 185–87

Dunne, J., K. Rebay-Salisbury, R. B. Salisbury, A. Frisch, C. Walton-Doyle, and R. P. Evershed, 'Milk of Ruminants in Ceramic Baby Bottles from Prehistoric Child Graves', *Nature*, 574.7777 (2019), 246–48

DuPuis, E. Melanie, *Nature's Perfect Food: How Milk Became America's Drink* (New York: New York University Press, 2002)

Elliott, Katherine, and David W. FitzSimons, *Breast-Feeding and the Mother* (Somerset, UK: John Wiley & Sons, Incorporated, 1976)

Emecheta, Buchi, *The Joys of Motherhood* (Heinemann, 1979)

Empson, Rebecca M., *Harnessing Fortune: Personhood, Memory and Place in Mongolia* (Oxford University Press, 2011)

Engelmajer, Pascale F., '"Like a Mother Her Only Child": Mothering in the Pāli Canon', *Open Theology*, 6.1 (2020), 88–103

Ehrenreich, Barbara, and Deirdre English, *Witches, Midwives and Nurses: A History of Women Healers*, 2nd edn (New York: Feminist Press at City University of New York, 2010)

Epstein-Gilboa, Keren, 'Breastfeeding Envy: Unresolved Patriarchal Envy and the Obstruction of Physiologically-Based Nursing Patterns', in *Giving Breastmilk: Body Ethics and Contemporary Breastfeeding Practices*, eds Rhonda Shaw and Alison Bartlett (Toronto: Demeter Press, 2010)

Falls, Susan, *White Gold: Stories of Breast Milk Sharing* (Lincoln, US: Nebraska, 2017)

Fildes, Valerie, *Breasts, Bottles, and Babies* (Edinburgh: Edinburgh University Press, 1986)

———, 'The Culture and Biology of Breastfeeding: An Historical Review of Western Europe', in *Breastfeeding: Biocultural Perspectives* (Routledge, 1995)

Filippini, Nadia Maria, *Pregnancy, Delivery, Childbirth: A Gender and Cultural History from Antiquity to the Test Tube in Europe* (Oxon: Routledge, 2021)

Filson, Jon, 'Taste Test', *Toronto Star*, 14 July 2006

Forbes, Gordon B., Leah E. Adams-Curtis, Nicole R. Hamm, and Kay B. White, 'Perceptions of the Woman Who Breastfeeds: The Role of Erotophobia, Sexism, and Attitudinal Variables', *Sex Roles*, 49.7/8 (2003), 379–88

Frampton, Edith, 'Fluid Objects: Kleinian Psychoanalytic Theory and Breastfeeding Narratives', *Australian Feminist Studies*, 19.45 (2004), 357–68

———, '"Writing in White Ink": Reconfiguring the Body of the Wet Nurse', in *Back to the Future of the Body*, ed. Dominic Janes (Cambridge Scholars Publishing, 2007)

Gaard, Greta, 'Toward a Feminist Postcolonial Milk Studies', *American Quarterly*, 65.3 (2013), 595–618

Giladi, Avner, *Infants, Parents and Wet Nurses: Medieval Islamic Views on Breastfeeding and Their Social Implications* (Leiden: Brill, 1999)

Giles, Fiona, '"Relational, and Strange": A Preliminary Foray into a Project to Queer Breastfeeding', *Australian Feminist Studies*, 19.45 (2004), 301–314

———, *The Secret Life of Breasts* (New York: Simon & Schuster, 2003)

———, 'The Tears of Lacteros: Integrating the Meanings of the Human Breast', in *Body Parts: Critical Explorations in Corporeality*, eds Christopher E. Forth and Ivan Crozier (Lexington Books, 2005), pp. 123–41

———, 'The Uses Of Pleasure: Reconfiguring Lactation, Sexuality and Mothering', in *Theorising and Representing Maternal Realities*, eds Marie Porter and Julie Kelso (Cambridge Scholars Publishing, 2008), pp. 21–37

Granheim, S. I., Katrin Engelhardt, P. Rundall, S. Bialous, Alessandro D. Iellamo, and B. Margetts, 'Interference in Public Health Policy: Examples of How the Baby Food Industry Uses Tobacco Industry Tactics', 2017

Grayson, Jennifer, *Unlatched: The Evolution of Breastfeeding and the Making of a Controversy* (New York: Harper, 2016)

Green, Monica, *Making Women's Medicine Masculine: The Rise of Male Authority in Pre-Modern Gynaecology* (Oxford: Oxford University Press, 2008)

Griffiths, Jay, *Pip Pip: A Sideways Look at Time* (London: HarperPress, 2000)

Grig, Lucy, 'Portraits, Pontiffs and the Christianization of Fourth-Century Rome', *Papers of the British School at Rome*, 72 (2004), 203–30

Guillemeau, Jacques, *Child-Birth or, The Happy Delivery of Vvomen* (London: Printed by Anne Griffin, for Ioyce Norton, and Richard Whitaker, 1635)

Haga Gripsrud, Birgitta, 'The Cultural History of the Breast', in *Cultural Encyclopedia of the Body* (Greenwood Publishing, 2008), I, 31–44

Haga Gripsrud, Birgitta, Ellen Ramvi, Lynn Froggett, Ingvil Hellstrand, and Julian Manley, 'Psychosocial and Symbolic Dimensions of the Breast Explored through a Visual Matrix', *NORA – Nordic Journal of Feminist and Gender Research*, 26.3 (2018), 210–29

Hall, D. M. B., 'Tongue Tie', *Archives of Disease in Childhood*, 90.12 (2005), 1211–15

Hamilton, Lucy Phelps, '"If De Babies Cried": Slave Motherhood in Antebellum Missouri' (unpublished masters dissertation, Pittsburg State University, 2015)

Harley, David, 'From Providence to Nature: The Moral Theology and Godly Practice of Maternal Breast-Feeding in Stuart England', *Bulletin of the History of Medicine*, 69.2 (1995), 198–223

Harraway, Donna, 'Situated Knowledges: The Science Question in Feminism and the Privilege of Partial Perspective', *Feminist Studies*, 14.3 (1988), 575–99

Hastings, Gerard, Kathryn Angus, Douglas Eadie, and Kate Hunt, 'Selling Second Best: How Infant Formula Marketing Works', *Globalization and Health*, 16.1 (2020), 77

Hastrup, Kirsten, 'A Question of Reason: Brest-Feeding Patterns in Seventeenth- and Eighteenth-Century Iceland', in *The Anthropology of Breast-Feeding*, ed. Vanessa Maher (Oxford: Berg, 1992), pp. 91–108

Hausman, Bernice, 'The Feminist Politics of Breastfeeding', *Australian Feminist Studies*, 19.45 (2004), 273–85

Havard, Lucy Ann, 'Kahlo, Mexicanidad and Máscaras: The Search for Identity in Postcolonial Mexico', *Romance Studies*, 24.3 (2006), 241–51

Hebron, Micol, 'Reviews: Separation Anxiety', *Art Pulse* http://artpulsemagazine.com/separation-anxiety [accessed 7 November 2021]

Heise, Alia, and Diane Wiessinger, 'Dysphoric Milk Ejection Reflex: A Case Report', *International Breastfeeding Journal*, 6 (2011), 6

Hermanson Meister, Sarah, *Dorothea Lange: Migrant Mother* (New York: The Museum of Modern Art, 2018)

Herrera, Hayden, *Frida* (London: Bloomsbury, 2003)

Hewlett, Barry S., and Steve Winn, 'Allomaternal Nursing in Humans', *Current Anthropology*, 55.2 (2014), 200–229

Hill Collins, Patricia, 'Shifting the Center: Race, Class, and Feminist Theorizing about Motherhood', in *Representations of Motherhood*, eds Donna Bassin, Meryle Mahrer Kaplan, and Margaret Honey (Yale University Press, 1996)

Hill, Marsha, 'Nursing Women', in *Egyptian Art in the Age of the Pyramids* (New York: Metropolitan Museum of Art, 1999), pp. 393–94

Hinde, Katie, Amy L. Skibiel, Alison B. Foster, Laura Del Rosso, Sally P. Mendoza, and John P. Capitanio, 'Cortisol in Mother's Milk across Lactation Reflects Maternal Life History and Predicts Infant Temperament', *Behavioral Ecology*, 26.1 (2014), 269–81

Hoban, E., 'We're Safe and Happy Already: Traditional Birth Attendants and Safe Motherhood in a Cambodian Rural Commune' (unpublished PhD thesis, The University of Melbourne, 2002)

Hoffkling, Alexis, Juno Obedin-Maliver, and Jae Sevelius, 'From Erasure to Opportunity: A Qualitative Study of the Experiences of Transgender Men around Pregnancy and Recommendations for Providers', *BMC Pregnancy and Childbirth*, 17.2 (2017), 332

Hoffman, Kelly M., Sophie Trawalter, Jordan R. Axt, and M. Norman Oliver, 'Racial Bias in Pain Assessment and Treatment Recommendations, and False Beliefs about Biological

Differences between Blacks and Whites', *Proceedings of the National Academy of Sciences of the United States of America*, 113.16 (2016), 4296–301

hooks, bell, *Feminist Theory: From Margin to Center* (South End Press, 1984)

Horsley, Ritta Jo, and Richard A. Horsley, 'On the Trail of the "Witches": Wise Women, Midwives and the European Witch Hunts', *Women in German Yearbook*, 3 (1987), 1–28

Hudson, P., and W. R. Lee, eds, *Women's Work and the Family Economy in Historical Perspective* (Manchester: Manchester University Press, 1990)

Jacobsen, Knut A., 'The Child Manifestation of Śiva in Contemporary Hindu Popular Prints', *Numen*, 51.3 (2004), 237–64

Jacobus, M. L., 'Incorruptible Milk: Breast-Feeding and the French Revolution', in *Rebel Daughters – Women and the French Revolution* (Oxford University Press, 1992), pp. 54–78.

Jakobson, R., 'Why "Mama" and "Papa"?', in *Readings in Modern Linguistics: An Anthology* (De Gruyter Mouton, 2019), pp. 313–20

Johnson, Clare, and Jenny Rintoul, 'From Nursing Virgins to Belfries: The Project of Maternal Femininity', *Journal of Gender Studies*, 28.8 (2019), 918–36

Jones, Vivien, 'The Death of Mary Wollstonecraft', *Journal for Eighteenth-Century Studies*, 20.2 (1997), 187–205

Juneja, Monica, 'The Breastfeeding Mother as Icon and Source of Affect in Visual Practice – A Transcultural Journey', in *Looking Within Looking Without: Exploring Households in the Subcontinent Through Time*, ed. Kumkum Roy (Delhi: Primus Books, 2015), pp. 105–36

Kassam, Ashifa, 'Breastfeeding as a Trans Dad: "A Baby Doesn't Know What Your Pronouns Are"', *Guardian*, 20 June 2016, https://www.theguardian.com/society/2016/jun/20/transgender-dad-breastfeeding-pregnancy-trevor-macdonald [accessed 27 September 2021]

Kateusz, Ally, *Mary and Early Christian Women* (Palgrave Macmillan, 2019)

Kessen, William, 'Rousseau's Children', *Daedalus*, 107.3 (1978), 155–66

Kinsella, Tina, 'Querying and Queering the Virgin: Iconography and Iconoclasticism in the Art of Frida Kahlo', *Tina Kinsella*, 2011

Kintner, Hallie J., 'Trends and Regional Differences in Breast-feeding in Germany From 1871 To 1937', *Journal of Family History*, 10.2 (1985), 163–82

Kipp, Julie, *Romanticism, Maternity, and the Body Politic* (Cambridge University Press, 2003)

Knight, K., K. Bunch, D. Tuffnell, R. Patel, J. Shakespeare, R. Kotnis, and others, *Saving Lives, Improving Mothers' Care – Lessons Learned to Inform Maternity Care from the UK and Ireland Confidential Enquiries into Maternal Deaths and Morbidity 2017–19* (Oxford: National Perinatal Epidemiology Unit, University of Oxford, 2021)

Knodel, John, and Etienne Van de Walle, 'Breast Feeding, Fertility and Infant Mortality: An Analysis of Some Early German Data', *Population Studies*, 21.2 (1967), 109–31

Kozol, Wendy, 'Domesticating NATO's War in Kosovo/a: (In) Visible Bodies and the Dilemma of Photojournalism', *Meridians*, 4.2 (2004), 1–38

Kristeva, Julia, *Powers of Horror* (New York: Columbia University Press, 1982)

Krögel, Alison, 'Mercenary Milk, Pernicious Nursemaids, Heedless Mothers: Anti-Wet Nurse Rhetoric in the Satirical Ordenanzas Del Baratillo de Mexico (1734)', *Dieciocho: Hispanic Enlightenment*, 37.2 (2014)

Kukla, Rebecca, 'Ethics and Ideology in Breastfeeding Advocacy Campaigns', *Hypatia*, 21.1 (2006), 157–80

Labbok, Miriam, *Exploration of Guilt Among Mothers Who Do Not Breastfeed: The Physician's Role*, 2008, XXIV

Laroia, Nirupama, and Deeksha Sharma, 'The Religious and Cultural Bases for Breastfeeding Practices Among the Hindus', *Breastfeeding Medicine*, 1.2 (2006), 94–98

Lavely, William, 'Sex, Breastfeeding, and Marital Fertility in Pre-transition China', *Population and Development Review*, 33.2 (2007), 289–320

Leslie, Esther, and Melanie Jackson, 'Milk's Arrays', *Studies in the Maternal*, 10.1 (2018)

Levene, Alysa, 'The Estimation of Mortality at the London Foundling Hospital, 1741–99', *Population Studies*, 59.1 (2005), 87–97

Levy, Ariel, 'Catherine Opie, All-American Subversive', *The New Yorker*, 13 March 2017, https://www.newyorker.com/magazine/

2017/03/13/catherine-opie-all-american-subversive?utm_ source=NYR_REG_GATE [accessed 3 March 2021]

Leyser, Henrietta, *Medieval Women: Social History Of Women In England 450–1500* (W&N, 2005)

Liamputtong, Pranee, *Childrearing and Infant Care Issues: A Cross-Cultural Perspective* (Nova Publishers, 2007)

Liscio, Lorraine, 'Beloved's Narrative: Writing Mother's Milk', *Tulsa Studies in Women's Literature*, 11.1 (1992), 31–46

Liss, Andrea, *Feminist Art and the Maternal* (University of Minnesota Press, 2009)

Littler, Jo, 'Mothers Behaving Badly: Chaotic Hedonism and the Crisis of Neoliberal Social Reproduction', *Cultural Studies*, 34.4 (2020), 499–520

Lyon, J. Vanessa, 'Full of Grace: Lactation, Expression and "Colorito" Painting in Some Early Works by Rubens', in *Medieval and Renaissance Lactations*, ed. Jutta Gisela Sperling (Routledge, 2013)

MacDonald, Trevor, *Where's the Mother?: Stories from a Transgender Dad* (Trans Canada Press, 2016).

MacDonald, Trevor, Joy Noel-Weiss, Diana West, Michelle Walks, MaryLynne Biener, Alanna Kibbe, and others, 'Transmasculine Individuals' Experiences with Lactation, Chestfeeding, and Gender Identity: A Qualitative Study', *BMC Pregnancy and Childbirth*, 16.1 (2016), 106

MacLeod, K. J., and D. Lukas, 'Revisiting Non-Offspring Nursing: Allonursing Evolves When the Costs Are Low', *Biology Letters*, 10.6 (2014), 20140378

Maher, Vanessa, 'Breast-Feeding and Maternal Depletion: Natural Law or Cultural Arrangements?', in *The Anthropology of Breast-Feeding*, ed. Vanessa Maher (Berg, 1992), pp. 151–80

———, 'Breast-Feeding in Cross-Cultural Perspective: Paradoxes and Proposals', in *The Anthropology of Breast-Feeding*, ed. Vanessa Maher (Oxford: Berg, 1992), pp. 1–36

———, ed., *The Anthropology of Breast-Feeding: Natural Law or Social Construct* (Oxford: Berg, 1992)

Marshall, C. W., 'Breastfeeding in Greek Literature and Thought', *Illinois Classical Studies*, 42.1 (2017), 185–201

Maryline Parca, 'The Wet Nurses of Ptolemaic and Roman Egypt', *Illinois Classical Studies*, 42.1 (2017), 203–26

Mazzoni, Cristina, *She-Wolf: The Story of a Roman Icon* (Cambridge University Press, 2010)

McClure, Ruth K., *Coram's Children: The London Foundling Hospital in the Eighteenth Century* (New Haven: Yale University Press, 1981)

Mccoid, Catherine Hodge, Leroy D. Mcdermott, 'Toward Decolonizing Gender', *American Anthropologist*, 98.2 (1996), 319–26

Męcińska, Aleksandra Maria, 'Social Struggles Over Breastfeeding: How Lactivism Reshapes Knowledge, Meanings, And Practices Of Breastfeeding.' (unpublished PhD thesis, Lancaster University, 2017)

Mendham, Matthew D., 'Rousseau's Discarded Children: The Panoply of Excuses and the Question of Hypocrisy', *History of European Ideas*, 41.1 (2015), 131–52

Mitchell, Les, *Reading the Animal Text in the Landscape of the Damned* (NISC (Pty) Ltd, 2019)

Mock, Michele, 'Spitting out the Seed: Ownership of Mother, Child, Breasts, Milk, and Voice in Toni Morrison's *Beloved*, *College Literature*, 23.3 (1996), 117–26

Morgan, Jennifer L., '"Some Could Suckle over Their Shoulder": Male Travelers, Female Bodies, and the Gendering of Racial Ideology, 1500-1770', *The William and Mary Quarterly*, 54.1 (1997), 167–92

'Mothers Told "Breast Milk Is Best"', *BBC News*, 17 May 1999 http://news.bbc.co.uk/1/hi/health/345693.stm [accessed 25 November 2021]

Murphy, E. M., '"The Child That Is Born of One's Fair Body" – Maternal and Infant Death in Medieval Ireland', *Childhood in the Past*, 14.1 (2021), 13–37

Nakayama, Izumi, '3. Moral Responsibility for Nutritional Milk: Motherhood and Breastfeeding in Modern Japan', eds Angela Ki Che Leung, Melissa L. Caldwell, Robert Ji-Song Ku, and Christine R. Yano (University of Hawaii Press, 2020), pp. 66–88

Obladen, Michael, 'Pap, Gruel, and Panada: Early Approaches to Artificial Infant Feeding', *Neonatology*, 105.4 (2014), 267–74

OECD and World Health Organization, *Health at a Glance: Asia/Pacific 2020: Measuring Progress Towards Universal Health Coverage*, (OECD, 2020)

Ohaja, Magdalena, and Chinemerem Anyim, 'Rituals and Embodied Cultural Practices at the Beginning of Life: African Perspectives', *Religions*, 12.11 (2021)

Ohnuma, Reiko, *Ties That Bind: Maternal Imagery and Discourse in Indian Buddhism* (Oxford: Oxford University Press, 2012)

Omari-Tunkara, Mikelle Smith, *Manipulating the Sacred: Yorùbá Art, Ritual, and Resistance in Brazilian Candomblé* (Wayne State University Press, 2006)

O'Reilly, Andrea, 'Matricentric Feminism: A Feminism for Mothers', *Journal of the Motherhood Initiative*, 10.1–2 (2019)

Orland, Barbara, 'Why Could Early Modern Men Lactate? Gender Identity and Metabolic Narrations in Humoral Medicine.', in *Medieval and Renaissance Lactations*, ed. Jutta Gisela Sperling (Routledge, 2013)

Otero, Solimar, and Toyin Falola, eds., *Yemoja: Gender, Sexuality, and Creativity in the Latina/o and Afro-Atlantic Diasporas* (State University of New York Press, 2013)

Painter, Nell Irvin, 'Representing Truth: Sojourner Truth's Knowing and Becoming Known.', *The Journal of American History*, 81.2 (1994), 461–92

Palmer, Gabrielle, *The Politics of Breastfeeding. When Breasts Are Bad for Business*, 3rd edn (Pinter and Martin, 2009)

Pedrucci, Giulia, 'Breastfeeding Animals and Other Wild "Nurses" in Greek and Roman Mythology', *Gerión. Revista de Historia Antigua*, 34 (2016)

———, 'Kourotrophia and "Mothering" Figures: Conceiving and Raising an Infant as a Collective Process in the Greek, Etruscan, and Roman Worlds. Some Religious Evidences in Narratives and Art', *Open Theology*, 6.1 (2020), 145–66

Pelto, Gretel H., 'Perspectives on Infant Feeding: Decision-Making and Ecology', *Food and Nutrition Bulletin*, 3.3 (1981), 1–15

Pereira-Kotze, Catherine, Bill Jeffery, Jane Badham, Elizabeth C. Swart, Lisanne du Plessis, Ameena Goga, and others, 'Conflicts of Interest Are Harming Maternal and Child Health: Time for Scientific Journals to End Relationships with Manufacturers of Breast-Milk Substitutes', *BMJ Global Health*, 7.2 (2022), e008002

Perkins, Wendy, *Midwifery And Medicine In Early Modern France: Louise Bourgeois* (Exeter: University of Exeter Press, 1996)

Perry, Ruth, 'Colonizing the Breast: Sexuality and Maternity in Eighteenth-Century England', *Journal of the History of Sexuality*, 2.2 (1991), 204–34

Pfeufer Kahn, Robbie, 'Women and Time in Childbirth and During Lactation', in *Feminist Perspectives on Temporality*, eds Frieda Johles Forman and Caoran Sowton (Oxford: Pergamon Press, 1988), pp. 20–36

Piwoz, Ellen G., and Sandra L. Huffman, 'The Impact of Marketing of Breast-Milk Substitutes on WHO-Recommended Breastfeeding Practices', *Food and Nutrition Bulletin*, 36.4 (2015), 373–86

Plutarch, Moralia, *Volume VII: On Love of Wealth. On Compliancy. On Envy and Hate. On Praising Oneself Inoffensively. On the Delays of the Divine Vengeance. On Fate. On the Sign of Socrates. On Exile. Consolation to His Wife*, trans. Phillip H. de Lacey and Benedict Einarson (Cambridge MA: Harvard University Press, 1959)

Pollock, Griselda, *Mary Cassatt: Painter of Modern Women* (London: Thames and Hudson, 1998)

———, *Vision and Difference: Femininity, Feminism, and the Histories of Art* (London: Routledge, 1988)

Polomeno, Viola, 'Sex and Breastfeeding: An Educational Perspective', *The Journal of Perinatal Education*, 8.1 (1999), 30–40

Price, Theodora Hadzisteliou, *Kourotrophos: Cults and Representations of the Greek Nursing Deities* (Brill Archive, 1978)

Raynalde, Thomas, *The Birth of Mankind: Otherwise Named, The Woman's Book : Newly Set Forth, Corrected, and Augmented : Whose Contents Ye May Read in the Table of the Book, and Most Plainly in the Prologue / [Eucharius Rösslin] ; [Revised and Augmented] by Thomas Reynalde, Physician, 1560*, ed. Elaine Hobby (Ashgate, 2009)

Reisman, Tamar, and Zil Goldstein, 'Case Report: Induced Lactation in a Transgender Woman', *Transgender Health*, 3.1 (2018), 24–26

Rendle-Short, J., 'William Cadogan, Eighteenth-Century Physician', *Medical History*, 4.4 (1960), 288–309

Renfrew, Mary J., *Preventing Disease and Saving Resources: The Potential Contribution of Increasing Breastfeeding Rates in the UK* (UNICEF)

Rich, Adrienne, *Of Woman Born: Motherhood as an Experience and Institution* (New York: Norton, 1986)

Roehrig, Catharine H., 'Women's Work: Some Occupations of Non-Royal Women as Depicted in Ancient Egyptian Art', in *Mistress of the House, Mistress of Heaven: Women in Ancient Egypt*, eds Anne K. Capel and Glenn E. Markoe (New York: Hudson Hills Press, 1996)

Rollins, Nigel C., Nita Bhandari, Nemat Hajeebhoy, Susan Horton, Chessa K. Lutter, Jose C. Martines, and others, 'Why Invest, and What It Will Take to Improve Breastfeeding Practices?', *The Lancet*, 387.10017 (2016), 491–504

Roulin, Jean-Marie, 'Mothers in Revolution: Political Representations of Maternity in Nineteenth-Century France', *Yale French Studies*, 101 (2001), 182–200

Rowold, Katharina, 'Modern Mothers, Modern Babies: Breastfeeding and Mother's Milk in Interwar Britain', *Women's History Review*, 28 (2019), 1–20

———, 'Other Mothers' Milk: From Wet Nursing to Human Milk Banking in England, 1900-1950', *Cultural and Social History*, 16.5 (2019), 603–20

Ryan, Kieran, 'Manhood and the "Milk of Human Kindness" in *Macbeth*', *The British Library*, 2016, https://www.bl.uk/shakespeare/articles/manhood-and-the-milk-of-human-kindness-in-macbeth [accessed 16 July 2021]

Salmon, Marylynn, 'The Cultural Significance of Breastfeeding and Infant Care in Early Modern England and America', *Journal of Social History*, 28.2 (1994), 247–69

Sánchez Romero, Margarita, and Rosa López, 'Motherhood and Infancies: Archaeological and Historical Approaches', in *Motherhood and Infancies in the Mediterranean in Antiquity*, 2018, pp. 1–11

Sayej, Nadja, 'Cindy Sherman and Catherine Opie Make a Strangely Charming Cameo in Jewelry Together', *W Magazine*, 2019, https://www.wmagazine.com/story/cindy-sherman-catherine-opie-cameo-lizworks-jewelry [accessed 20 October 2021]

Schiebinger, Londa, 'Why Mammals Are Called Mammals: Gender Politics in Eighteenth-Century Natural History', *The American Historical Review*, 98.2 (1993), 382–411

Seals Allers, Kimberly, *The Big Letdown: How Medicine, Big Business, and Feminism Undermine Breastfeeding* (New York: St Martin's Press, 2016)

Seaman, Kristen, *Rhetoric and Innovation in Hellenistic Art* (Cambridge: University of Cambridge Press, 2020)

Segawa, Masashi, 'Buddhism and Breastfeeding', *Breastfeeding Medicine*, 3.2 (2008), 124–28

Selby, Martha Ann, 'Women as Patients and Practitioners in Early Sanskrit Medical Literature', in *Looking Within Looking Without: Exploring Households in the Subcontinent Through Time*, ed. Kumkum Roy (Delhi: Primus Books, 2015), pp. 49–73

Senior, Nancy, 'Aspects of Infant Feeding in Eighteenth-Century France', *Eighteenth-Century Studies*, 16.4 (1983), 367–88

Shaw, Rhonda, 'The Virtues of Cross-Nursing and the "yuk Factor"', Australian Feminist Studies, 19.45 (2004), 287–99

Shorter, Edward, *The Making of the Modern Family* (Fontana Books, 1979)

Smith, Hugh, *Letters to Married Women on Nursing and the Management of Children*, 2nd edn (Philadephia: Mathew Carey, 1796)

Soto, Ana, Virginia Martín, Esther Jiménez, Isabelle Mader, Juan M Rodríguez, and Leonides Fernández, 'Lactobacilli and Bifidobacteria in Human Breast Milk: Influence of Antibiotherapy and Other Host and Clinical Factors', *Journal of Pediatric Gastroenterology and Nutrition*, 59.1 (2014), 78–88

Spagnoletti, Belinda Rina Marie, Linda Rae Bennett, Michelle Kermode, and Siswanto Agus Wilopo, 'Moralising Rhetoric and Imperfect Realities: Breastfeeding Promotions and the Experiences of Recently Delivered Mothers in Urban Yogyakarta, Indonesia', *Asian Studies Review*, 42.1 (2018), 17–38

Sparey, Victoria, 'Breastfeeding Mothers and Milk in Shakespeare', *Early Modern Medicine*, 2013

———, 'Identity-Formation and the Breastfeeding Mother in Renaissance Generative Discourses and Shakespeare's *Coriolanus*', *Social History of Medicine*, 25.4 (2012), 777–94

Sperling, Jutta Gisela, *Medieval and Renaissance Lactations Images, Rhetorics, Practices* (Routledge, 2013)

———, *Roman Charity: Queer Lactations in Early Modern Visual Culture* (Transcript Verlag, 2016)

Spivak, Gayatri Chakravorty, 'Introduction', in *Breast Stories* (New York: Seagull, 2018)

Stantis, Chris, Holger Schutkowski, and Arkadiusz Sołtysiak, 'Reconstructing Breastfeeding and Weaning Practices in the Bronze Age Near East Using Stable Nitrogen Isotopes', *American Journal of Physical Anthropology*, 172.1 (2020), 58–69

Steele, Cassie Premo, 'Drawing Strength from Our Mothers Tapping the Roots of Black Women's History', *Journal of the Motherhood Initiative for Research and Community Involvement*, 2.2 (2000)

Stephens, William, 'Lactile Libations: Mongolian Milk Offerings', *Missiology*, 49.1 (2021), 39–53

Stevens, Emily E., Thelma E. Patrick, and Rita Pickler, 'A History of Infant Feeding', *Journal of Perinatal Education*, 18.2 (2009), 32–39

Stone, Lawrence, *The Family, Sex and Marriage in England 1500-1800* (Pelican Books, 1979)

Strother, Z. S., 'A Terrifying Mimesis: Problems of Portraiture and Representation in African Sculpture (Congo-Kinshasa)', *Res: Anthropology and Aesthetics*, 65–66 (2015), 128–47

Stuart-Macadam, Patricia, 'Breastfeeding in Prehistory', in *Breastfeeding: Biocultural Perspectives*, eds Patricia Stuart-Macadam and Katherine A. Dettwyler (New York: Aldine de Gruyter, 1995), pp. 75–98

Suskin Ostriker, Alicia, *The Mother/Child Papers* (University of Pittsburgh Press, 2009)

Suśruta, and Kaviraj Kunjalal Bhishagratna, *An English Translation of the Sushruta Samhita Based on Original Sanskrit Text.* (Varanasi: Chowkhamba Sanskrit Series Office, 1981)

Sussman, George D., 'The Wet-Nursing Business in Nineteenth-Century France', *French Historical Studies*, 9.2 (1975), 304–28

Sweney, Mark, 'Mums Furious as Facebook Removes Breastfeeding Photos', *Guardian*, 30 December 2008, section Technology, https://www.theguardian.com/media/2008/dec/30/facebook-breastfeeding-ban [accessed 27 November 2021]

Tapper, Josh, 'Transgender Man Can Be Breastfeeding Coach', *Toronto Star*, 25 April 2014, section Health & Wellness, https://www.thestar.com/life/health_wellness/2014/04/25/transgender_man_can_be_breastfeeding_coach.html [accessed 20 November 2021].

—— 'La Leche League Canada Rejects Breastfeeding Dad's Bid to Become Lactation Coach', *Toronto Star*, 19

August 2012, section Canada, https://www.thestar.com/news/canada/2012/08/19/la_leche_league_canada_rejects_breastfeeding_dads_bid_to_become_lactation_coach.html [accessed 20 November 2021].

Tate, Carolyn. E., *Reconsidering Olmec Visual Culture. The Unborn, Women, and Creation* (University of Texas Press, 2012)

Thomson, Gill, Katherine Ebisch-Burton, and Renee Flacking, 'Shame If You Do – Shame If You Don't': Women's Experiences of Infant Feeding', *Maternal & Child Nutrition*, 11.1 (2015), 33–46

'Thousands Protest in Support of Breastfeeding "Tramp"', *BBC News*, 15 March 2014, section Stoke & Staffordshire, https://www.bbc.com/news/uk-england-stoke-staffordshire-26592340 [accessed 3 November 2021]

Toronchuk, J. A., and G. F. R. Ellis, 'Disgust: Sensory Affect or Primary Emotional System?', *Cognition and Emotion*, 21 (2007)

Totelin, Laurence, 'Milky Love', *Concoctinghistory*, 2013, https://ancientrecipes.wordpress.com/2013/07/12/milky-love [accessed 15 July 2021]

———, 'Of Milk and Honey', *Concoctinghistory*, 2013, https://ancientrecipes.wordpress.com/2013/05/14/of-milk-and-honey [accessed 15 July 2021]

———, 'Of Milk and Honey II', *Concoctinghistory*, 2013, https://ancientrecipes.wordpress.com/2013/05/30/of-milk-and-honey-ii [accessed 15 July 2021]

Trautner, Emily, Megan McCool-Myers, and Andrea Braden Joyner, 'Knowledge and Practice of Induction of Lactation in Trans Women among Professionals Working in Trans Health', *International Breastfeeding Journal*, 15.1 (2020), 63

Treckel, Paula A., 'Breastfeeding and Maternal Sexuality in Colonial America', *The Journal of Interdisciplinary History*, 20.1 (1989), 25–51

Tyebally Fang, Mirriam, Efstratios Chatzixiros, Laurence Grummer-Strawn, Cyril Engmann, Kiersten Israel-Ballard, Kimberly Mansen, and others, 'Developing Global Guidance on Human Milk Banking', *Bulletin of the World Health Organization*, 99.12 (2021), 892–900

UNICEF, and WHO, 'Nurturing the Health and Wealth of Nations: The Investment Case for Breastfeeding', 2017, https://www.who.int/nutrition/publications/infantfeeding/global-bf-collective-investmentcase.pdf?ua=1 [accessed 24 September 2021]

Valerius Maximus, *Memorable Words and Deeds*, trans. Henry John Walker (Indianapolis, 2004)

Van Esterik, Penny, 'Breast-Feeding as Food Work', in *Food and Culture*, eds Penny Van Esterik, Caroline Counihan, and Alice Julier (Routledge, 2013)

———, 'Rice And Milk In Thai Buddhism: Symbolic And Social Values Of Basic Food Substances.', *Crossroads: An Interdisciplinary Journal of Southeast Asian Studies*, 2.1 (1984), 46–58

Ventura, Gal, *Maternal Breast-Feeding and Its Substitutes in Nineteenth-Century French Art*: (BRILL, 2018)

Viazzo, Pier Paolo, Maria Bortolotto, and Andrea Zanotto, 'Child Care, Infant Mortality and the Impact of Legislation: The Case of Florence's Foundling Hospital, 1840–1940', *Continuity and Change*, 9.2 (1994), 243–69

Virgo, Vanisha, 'Breastfeeding as a Black Woman in Modern Day UK', *Association of Breastfeeding Mothers*, https://abm.me.uk/breastfeeding-information/breastfeeding-as-a-black-woman [accessed 8 May 2021]

Wallace, William E., 'Michelangelo's Wet Nurse', *Arion: A Journal of Humanities and the Classics*, 17.2 (2009), 51–55

Walter, M, 'The Folklore of Breastfeeding', *Bulletin of the New York Academy of Medicine*, 51.7 (1975), 870–76

Watkinson, Marcelina, Craig Murray, and Jane Simpson, 'Maternal Experiences of Embodied Emotional Sensations during Breast Feeding: An Interpretative Phenomenological Analysis', *Midwifery*, 36 (2016), 53–60

Watson Andaya, Barbara, *The Flaming Womb: Repositioning Women in Early Modern Southeast Asia* (University of Hawaii Press, 2006)

West, Emily, and Emily Knight, 'Mothers' Milk: Slavery, Wet-Nursing, and Black and White Women in the Antebellum South', *Journal of Southern History*, 83 (2017), 37–68

West, Jennifer, 'White Columns', *Frieze*, 2008, https://web.archive.org/web/20100608093758/http://www.frieze.com/issue/review/jennifer_west [accessed 9 May 2021]

Widom, Wendy, 'Facebook & Instagram Are Censoring Motherhood, Says 4th Trimester Bodies Project', *CBS News Chicago*,

30 July 2014, https://www.cbsnews.com/chicago/news/4th-trimester-bodies-project-facebook-instagram [accessed 27 November 2021]

Wilson, Kristin J., *Others' Milk: The Potential of Exceptional Breastfeeding* (Rutgers University Press, 2018)

Wolf, Jacqueline H., '"Mercenary Hirelings" or "A Great Blessing"?: Doctors' and Mothers' Conflicted Perceptions of Wet Nurses and the Ramifications for Infant Feeding in Chicago, 1871–1961', *Journal of Social History*, 33.1 (1999), 97–120

Wong, Tessa, 'Cambodia Breast Milk: The Debate over Mothers Selling Milk', *BBC News*, 29 March 2017, https://www.bbc.com/news/world-asia-39414820 [accessed 20 June 2021]

Wye, Deborah, *Louise Bourgeois* (New York: Museum of Modern Art, 1982)

Yate, Zainab, *When Breastfeeding Sucks* (Pinter & Martin, 2020)

Young, Iris Marion, 'Breasted Experience', in *Throwing Like a Girl and Other Essays in Feminist Philosophy and Social Theory* (Indiana University Press, 1990), pp. 189–209

——, 'Pregnant Embodiment: Subjectivity and Alienation', in *Throwing Like a Girl and Other Essays in Feminist Philosophy and Social Theory* (Indiana University Press, 1990), pp. 160–76

——, 'Throwing Like a Girl: A Phenomenology of Feminine Body Comportment, Motility and Spatiality', in *Throwing Like a Girl and Other Essays in Feminist Philosophy and Social Theory* (Indiana University Press, 1990), pp. 141–59

Zarzycka, Marta, *Gendered Tropes in War Photography: Mothers, Mourners, Soldiers* (New York: Routledge, 2017)

Zatta, Claudia, 'Aristotle on "the Sweat of the Earth"', *Philosophia*, 48 (2018), 55–70

INDEX

ACKNOWLEDGEMENTS

It takes a village to write a book and there are many people who nurtured this book to fruition. Thank you to my fabulous agent, Jo Unwin, who 'got' the idea instantly and who carried me in my moments of doubt. To my fantastic editor Jenny Lord at W&N, thank you for your always-astute feedback, which helped refine the vision and sharpen my prose. And her team at W&N – Kate Moreton, Georgia Goodall, Alainna Hadjigeorgiou and Katie Moss. Thanks to Jacqui Lewis for her careful and rigorous copyedit, which improved the book immeasurably. I would have never had the confidence to draft a book proposal had it not been for Helen Babbs and Alice White at Wellcome Stories, who commissioned an early essay about breast-feeding which then became the basis for this book. And thank you to Karen Hall for offering generous feedback on a draft.

I could never hope to be comprehensive to all experiences and perspectives. Yet this book and my thinking were shaped by many conversations with parents and grown-up children, historical accounts that didn't make the edit, and discussions with experts in a variety of fields. Thank you in particular to Zainab Yate, Leah Hazard, Indie McDowell, Taey Iohe, Jess Dobkin, Charlotte McGuinness, Lisa Mann, Lisa Schoyer, Karen Schwenkmeyer, Rebecca Empson,

Katherine Cross, Scilla Landale and Sylvia Batchelor. You each generously gave up your time to share your expertise, thoughts and artistic practice with me. I am also especially grateful to those who trusted me with their intimate experiences during the research for this book, especially Nell, Katie, Katherine, Emily, Bethany, Enuma, Olivia, Irum, Becky, Sarah, Charlotte, Nash, and those who wished to remain entirely anonymous. Thanks always to Professor Ashley Thompson, who continues to have a profound influence on my thinking.

Thank you to the Society of Authors and the Authors' Foundation, who provided funding to support me as I completed the research and writing of this book. I owe a debt of gratitude to many librarians, archivists and curators, and I must pay specific thanks to everyone involved in digitising projects, from funding to the painstaking work of uploading and cataloguing museum collections, archives, diaries and so on. Your meticulous work meant I was able to continue my research during lockdown. And, more importantly, you have enabled materials to remain accessible to those unable to visit the physical collections.

I am incredibly fortunate to have a supportive, loving and hilarious extended network of family and friends. I first shared the idea for this book with my parents, Jan and Pete, when I was perhaps six weeks post-partum and slightly delirious, as they drove me and my son through the countryside in the hopes of us both having a nap. Deepest thanks to you both for your unwavering belief in me, and for the many hours of free childcare since. Special thanks to my one-in-a-million mother-in-law, Deryn, and my always-encouraging siblings Philippa and Mike – I'm lucky to have you. Annie Jael Kwan, our Zoom calls during the writing of this book were a highlight of my week, but I am very pleased we've returned to having in-person cocktails together. To

Helen Butlin and Birgitte Røeggen, I love you both dearly and I hope you know how much you mean to me.

None of this would have been possible without the support of my preternaturally patient husband, Eoin. Thank you for making me laugh every single day and for always thinking that writing a book was a completely sensible thing for me to do. And to our beautiful child – truly, I would do it all again a million times over for you.

ABOUT THE AUTHOR

Joanna Wolfarth is an art historian. Previously visiting lecturer in Southeast Asian Art at SOAS, University of London,
she is now lecturer in History of Art at The Open University.
Milk is her first book.